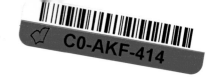

Springer Series on Epidemiology and Health

Series Editors
Wolfgang Ahrens
Iris Pigeot

For further volumes:
http://www.springer.com/series/7251

Jørn Olsen · Kaare Christensen · Jeff Murray ·
Anders Ekbom

An Introduction to Epidemiology for Health Professionals

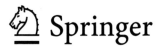

Jørn Olsen
School of Public Health
University of California, Los Angeles
Los Angeles CA 90095-1772
Box 951772
USA
jo@ucla.edu

Jeff Murray, MD
Department of Pediatrics
2182 MedLabs
University of Iowa
Iowa City, IA 52245
USA
jeff-murray@uiowa.edu

Kaare Christensen
Institute of Public Health
University of Southern Denmark
Sdr. Boulevard 23 A
5000 Odense C
Denmark
kchristensen@health.sdu.dk

Anders Ekbom
Department of Medicine,
  Karolinska Institute
SE-171 76 Stockholm
Sweden
anders.ekbom@ki.se

ISSN 1869-7933   e-ISSN 1869-7941
ISBN 978-1-4419-1496-5   e-ISBN 978-1-4419-1497-2
DOI 10.1007/978-1-4419-1497-2
Springer New York Dordrecht Heidelberg London

Library of Congress Control Number: 2010922282

Printed on acid-free paper

Springer is part of Springer Science+Business Media (www.springer.com)

Preface

There are many good epidemiology textbooks on the market, but most of these are addressed to students of public health or people who do clinical research with epidemiologic methods. There is a need for a short introduction on how epidemiologic methods are used in public health, genetic and clinical epidemiology, because health professionals need to know basic epidemiologic methods covering etiologic as well as prognostic factors of diseases. They need to know more about methodology than introductory texts on public health have to offer.

In some health faculties, epidemiology is not even part of the teaching curriculum. We believe this to be a serious mistake. Medical students are students of all aspects of diseases and health. Without knowing something about epidemiology the clinicians and other health professionals cannot read a growing part of the scientific literature in any reasonably critical way and cannot navigate in the world of "evidence-based medicine and evidence-based prevention." Without skills in epidemiologic methodology they are in the hands of experts that may not only have an interest in health.

Some health professionals may believe that only common sense is needed to conduct epidemiological studies, but the scientific literature and the public debate on health issues indicate that common sense is often in short supply and may not thrive without some formal training.

Epidemiologic methods play a key role in identifying environmental, social, and genetic determinants of diseases. Clinical epidemiology addresses the transition from disease to health or toward mortality or social or medical handicaps. Public health epidemiology addresses the transition from being healthy to being not healthy. Descriptive epidemiology provides the disease pattern that is needed to look at health in a broad perspective and to set the priorities right. Epidemiology is a basic science of medicine which addresses key questions such as "Who becomes ill?" and "What are important prognostic factors?" Answers to such questions provide the basis for better prevention and treatment of diseases.

Many people contributed to the writing of this book: medical students in Denmark, students of epidemiology at the IEA EEPE summer course in Florence, Italy, and students of public health in Los Angeles. Without technical assistance from Gitte Nielsen, Jenade Shelley, Nina Hohe and Pam Masangkay the book would never have materialized.

Los Angeles, California	Jørn Olsen
Odense, Denmark	Kaare Christensen
Iowa City, Iowa	Jeff Murray
Stockholm, Sweden	Anders Ekbom

Contents

A Short Introduction to Epidemiology

Epidemiology is an old scientific discipline that dates back to the middle of the nineteenth century. It is a discipline that aims at identifying the determinants of diseases and health in populations. It uses a population approach like demography, perhaps the scientific discipline that most closely resembles epidemiology. Epidemiology is defined by the object of research, "to identity determinants that change the occurrence of health phenomena in human populations."

Epidemiology is often associated with infectious diseases because an epidemic of a disease originally referred to an unexpected rise in the incidence of infectious diseases. Epidemiologic methods were first used to study diseases like cholera and measles. Now all diseases or health events are studied by means of epidemiologic methods and these methods are constantly changing to meet these new needs. Even the term "epidemic" is used to describe an unexpected increase in the frequency of any disease such as myocardial infarction, obesity, or asthma.

Today the discipline is used to study genetic, behavioral, and environmental causes of infectious and non-infectious diseases. The discipline is used to evaluate the effect of treatments or screening and it is the key discipline in the movement that may have been oversold with the title "evidence-based medicine."

Public health epidemiology uses the "healthy" population to study the transition from being healthy to being diseased or ill. Clinical epidemiology uses the population of patients to study predictors of cure or changes in the disease state. Both disciplines use experimental and non-experimental methods. Experimental methods are, however, often not applicable for ethical reasons in public health research since we cannot induce possibly harmful exposures on healthy people to address scientific hypotheses.

Epidemiologists have often been actors in political conflicts. Poverty, social inequalities, unemployment, and crowding are among the main determinants of health [1], and studying these determinants may bring epidemiologists into conflict with those who benefit from maintaining an unjust society. To some extent, these internal conflicts gave rise to clinical epidemiology. Many clinicians saw a need for using the methods developed in public health but did not like the idea of being associated with left-wing doctors fighting tuberculosis in India or poverty in Los Angeles. A clinical epidemiologist can study how best to treat diseases without taking an interest in how these diseases emerged.

We believe time has come to put an end to the artificial separation. Epidemiologists use the same set of tools and the same set of concepts whether they study the etiology or the prognosis of disease, although the methodological problems may reflect different circumstances. It is important to give priority to studying causal mechanisms that are amenable to intervention whether they affect prevention or treatment.

Epidemiology is among the basic medical sciences but is not quite recognized as such in many countries. Preventive medicine has been neglected by "patient-directed medicine" and been referred to specialists outside the clinical world. The process of evaluating new drugs has been left almost entirely to the pharmaceutical industry, not only to sponsor these studies but also to conduct and analyze the results.

Health professionals have to decide on treatments, perform diagnostic procedures, and give advice on prevention. This cannot be done without keeping an eye on the scientific literature, and at present a large part of what is published in medical journals is based on epidemiologic research. The same is true for much of the information that comes from pharmaceutical industries. Without some basic understanding of the limitations and sources of bias in this literature the clinician becomes a prisoner of his/her own ignorance; an easy victim of incorrect interpretations of data. Epidemiology may be the water that is needed in this desert of seduction.

Our intention has been to distill what is needed in the ordinary curriculum for health professionals who received an education without being exposed to epidemiologic textbooks. We present first a short introduction to the most common types of epidemiologic studies, how they are used, and their limitations. We then provide examples of how these methods have been used in public health, genetic epidemiology, and clinical research. Although each of these sub-disciplines has its own set of methods, most studies rely on the same basic set of logical reasoning. We leave out the statistical part of analyzing data and refer readers who take an interest in this to the many textbooks on this topic. We also refer readers to other textbooks to study the history of epidemiology [2]. Doing epidemiologic research requires following ethical standards and good practice rules for securing confidential data. We recommend reading the IEA guidelines on Good Epidemiologic Practice (www.ieaweb.org).

The book is short and condensed, but people in medical professions are clever and are trained in absorbing abstract information rapidly. Epidemiology is training in logical thinking rather than in memorization and we hope this book will be a pleasant journey into a mindset for later expansion and use. Keep in mind that an important part of learning is also to be able to identify what you do not know but should be aware of before you express your opinion.

References

1. Frank JP. Academic address on the people's misery: mother of all diseases. Bull Hist Med 1941 [first published 1790];9:88–100.
2. Holland WW, Olsen J, Florey CDV (eds.). Development of Epidemiology: Personal Reports from Those Who Were There. Oxford University Press, Oxford, 2007.

Part I
Descriptive Epidemiology

Chapter 1
Measures of Disease Occurrence

Setting priorities in public health planning for disease prevention depends on a set of conditions. Public health priorities should be set by the combination of how serious diseases are (a product of their frequency and the impact they have on those affected and society) and our ability to change their frequency or severity. This intervention requires knowledge of how to treat and/or to prevent the disease. If we have sufficient knowledge about the causes of the disease and if these causes are avoidable we may be able to propose effective preventive programs. If we do not have that knowledge research is needed, and if we know where to search for causes this research can be specifically targeted. If the disease can be treated at a low cost and with little risk, prevention need not be better than cure but often will be.

Clinical medicine may have a tendency to focus on rare but interesting diseases, whereas public health should focus on the big picture taking the frequency of disease into consideration. What are the possibilities of saving many lives, preventing ill health and social impairments with our available resources, and how do we best use these resources?

A number of measures are used to describe the frequency of a disease, but to begin with we could count the number of people with the disease in the population (the *prevalence* of the disease). We might also like to know how many new cases appear over a given time period either as an estimate of the risk of getting the disease over a given time span or as a rate, defined as new cases per time unit (the *cumulative incidence* or the *incidence rate*). We have to accept that we only estimate the force of morbidity, or mortality, in the population. We do not measure these parameters, but the quality of our estimates depends on how close we come to true parameters. When you start an investigation you want to know who the diseased are, when they got the disease, and where they live. "Who, when, and where" questions are the first questions you should ask.

Estimates of incidence (new cases) are needed to study the etiology of disease and to monitor preventive efforts. Monitoring programs of the incidence of cancer have, for example, been set up in many parts of the world and are being reported by IARC (The International Agency for Research on Cancer) in monographs like *Cancer Incidence in Five Continents* [1]. No other diseases have similar high-quality monitoring of incidence worldwide, but several routine registration systems

J. Olsen et al., *An Introduction to Epidemiology for Health Professionals*,
Springer Series on Epidemiology and Health 1, DOI 10.1007/978-1-4419-1497-2_1,
© Springer Science+Business Media, LLC 2010

for disease incidences exist in various parts of the world, either for total populations or for segments of the population. Many countries monitor, for example, incidences (new cases) of infectious diseases. Such monitoring systems rarely identify everybody with the infection and they need not cover all to pick up *epidemics* (unusual departures from average incidence rates that occur over shorter time spans). If a stable percentage is present over some period of time major fluctuations in the incidence of the disease in the population can be demonstrated. If very early markers of an epidemic are needed surrogate measures such as sales data of certain medication or the frequency of certain types of questions addressed to certain websites may even be useful.

Maternal, infant, and childhood mortality have been monitored in many parts of the world and they are often considered strong indicators of general health. Data on mortality are generally of good quality. Mortality is well defined and is not hampered by the ambiguous diagnosing that influences many disease registries where cause-specific mortality (disease-specific mortality or diseases that were proximal causes of the death) is measured.

Prevalence (existing cases at a given point in time) data are key in health planning. How many people do we have in our population with diabetes, multiple sclerosis, schizophrenia, etc.? How many and what kind of treatment facilities are needed to serve these people?

While incidence data can, in principle, be measured if we are able to define a set of operational diagnostic criteria, it may sometimes be more difficult to define prevalence (the number of diseased at a given point in time). For example, what is the prevalence of cancer? People who are treated successfully for cancer do not belong to the prevalent pool of diseased, but only time will tell whether the treatment cured the disease or not. In like manner, do people with asthma have the disease for the rest of their lives? Or people with epilepsy? Or people with type 2 diabetes or migraine? And if not, when are they cured? If we have no empirical data to identify people who leave the prevalent pool of cases, then our estimate of prevalence is difficult to interpret and use. It is easier with measles. When the signs of infection have disappeared and the virus can no longer be detected in the body, the person no longer has measles.

Incidence and Prevalence

A person may either have a disease, not have a disease, or have something in between. So when does a person become affected? In tallying diseases we need to use a set of criteria that indicates whether the person has the disease or not. For most diseases, we use a classification system like the International Classification of Diseases (ICD) [2] to force people into one group or the other. Over a lifetime each of us will get a given disease or we will not get the disease in question, but notice that this probability has a time dimension. If you die at the age of 30, you are less likely to suffer from a stroke in your lifetime than if you die at the age of 90.

For that reason, we expect many more cancer cases in developing countries if life expectancy continues to increase for these populations.

The risk of getting a disease is usually a function of time and these probabilities are estimated from the observation of populations. By observing the occurrence of diseases in populations over time we may be able to estimate incidence and prevalence of certain diseases. We use these estimates to compare disease occurrence between populations, to follow disease occurrence over time, and also to get an idea of disease risks for individuals in the population. To do this we will try to think about the population the person is part of; we will take gender, age, time, ethnic group, social conditions, place of residence, and information of other risk factors into consideration when we provide our estimate. For the individual such an estimate may be used to consider changes in behavior to modify, usually to reduce, this risk. But notice it is an indicator of risk, not a destiny. It is a prediction with uncertainty. In the end the person will either get the disease or not. If we say the person has a 25% risk of getting the disease within the next 10 years it does not mean that he/she will be 25% diseased. It means that among, say, 1,000 people with his/her characteristics we will expect about 250 to develop the disease. The person in question would like to know if he/she is among the 250 or not, but we will never be able to provide that information. We may, however, be able to make our predictions more informative, to make them closer to 0 or 100%. Many had hoped that the mapping of the human genome would bring us closer to predicting disease occurrence than it actually has except for a few specific diseases.

To estimate incidence and prevalence in a given population we need to identify the population and examine everyone in it, or a sample of them, at a given point in time (to estimate prevalence) or during a follow-up time period (to estimate incidence).

Assume we want to estimate the prevalence of type 1 diabetes in a city with 100,000 inhabitants. We may call them all in for a medical examination or we may base our estimate on a sample randomly selected from that population. Random selection implies, in its simplest form, that all members of the community have the same probability of being sampled. We could, for example, enumerate all inhabitants with a running number from 1 to 100,000. We could then select the first 10,000 random numbers and call them in for examination. Or we could draw a number at random from 0 to 9. Assuming that the number is 7, we could examine everybody in the population who had a running number ending with 7 (7, 17, 27, . . ., 99,997), which would also generate a sample of 10%. Or we could select everyone who was born on three randomly selected days in the month (say 3, 12, 28) and examine each person born on these days, which would generate a systematic sample of approximately 10%. If we are allowed to assume that the disease occurrence is independent of the days of birth this sample will produce results similar to what is found in a random sample, except for the random variation that is an unavoidable part of the selection process.

Assume that we examine 10,000 in the sample and find 50 with diabetes type 1, a disease characterized by a deficiency in the beta cells of the endocrine pancreas leading to a disturbance in glucose homeostasis. We would first have to develop a set of criteria that would define type 1 diabetes from the health examination. We would then say that the prevalence (P) in this population is 50 and the prevalence proportion (PP) is 50/10,000 or 0.005 or 0.5%. Should we estimate the prevalence proportion in the city at large our best estimate would still be 0.005, but we would know that another random sample may lead to a slightly different result due to sampling variation, and we would take this sampling variation into consideration when reporting. In reality, there would be many other sources of uncertainty than just the random sampling, such as measurement errors and selection bias related to invited people who did not come to the examination. All these uncertainties should be included in our uncertainty interval. Unfortunately, we do not at present have good tools to do that. A statistical estimate of 95% confidence limit will produce the following result:

$$P_{l,u} = 0.0048, 0.006$$

The exact interpretation of the *confidence limits* (CLs) may be debated, but one interpretation is that 95 out of 100 CLs will include the true prevalence assuming all sampling conditions are fulfilled.

In short, our estimate of the *prevalence proportion* (PP) is

$$PP = \frac{\text{Everybody with the disease in a given population at a given point in time}}{\text{Everybody in that population at that point in time}}$$

Incidence

In etiologic research we try to identify risk factors for disease occurrence and, in our search for these risk factors, we normally take an interest in new (incident) cases. We may, for example, like to know if the incidence of diabetes is increasing over time or how much the incidence is higher in obese than in non-obese people. To estimate incidence we need to observe the population we are going to study over time. Assume that as a point of departure we use the population we studied before, then after the initial screening we would have $10,000 - 50 = 9,950$ people without diabetes type 1. This is our *population at risk*; they are at risk of becoming incident (new) cases of type 1 diabetes during follow-up. Being at risk for being diagnosed with diabetes for the first time only means that the risk is not 0 (like it would be for prevalent cases).

The task would now be to identify all new cases of type 1 diabetes during follow-up in our population of 9,950 people. Ideally, we would examine everybody for diabetes at regular and short intervals, but this is not really an option in larger studies. We could, however, examine everybody at the end of follow-up and identify all new cases. If we have no loss to follow-up (no one died from other causes than diabetes, and no one left our study group (our cohort)), we could then estimate the cumulative incidence (an estimate of disease risk for a given follow-up time).

Assume that we had a 5-year time period of follow-up with no loss to follow-up and 10 new type 1 diabetes cases diagnosed at the examination at the end of follow-up, our estimate of the cumulative incidence (CI) would be 10/9,950 = 0.001. That would be our estimate of the disease risk in this population in a time period of 5 years.

Rates and Dynamic Populations

Since it is difficult to establish a fixed cohort to follow over time we usually study dynamic (open) *populations* in which persons enter our study at different time periods and leave it again over time (die, or leave our study for other reasons). We therefore have to use a measure that takes this variation in observation time into consideration. We do it by estimating incidence rates (IR), new cases of diabetes per time unit of observation (a measure of change in disease state as a function of time – like speed measures the distance traveled per unit time). In the previous cohort example we may assume we managed to follow up all 9,950 for 2 years. The 9,940 disease-free people each provide 2 observation years to our study, or 19,880 person-years, and if we assume that the 10 diseased on average provide 1 year of observation time the IR would be $10/19,890$ years $= 0.0005$ years^{-1} or 5 cases per 10,000 observation years. Again, this estimate would come with some uncertainty especially since the number of cases is small.

Although it may be possible in a fixed cohort to follow all cohort members over a shorter time period, it will not be possible for longer time periods. People will leave the study area, some may die, and some will refuse to remain in the study. These people are *censored* at the time they leave the study. All we know is that they did not get the disease when we had them under observation. Whether they got the disease after they were censored and before we ended the observation, we do not know. If we exclude these people from the cohort we overestimate the cumulative risk because we do not take into consideration their disease-free observation time. If we include them and consider them not diseased, also for the time where we did not have them under observation, we underestimate the risk if some got the disease after the time of censoring and before we closed the observation. To take all the observation time into consideration we have to use the incidence rate, although we still face the problem that the censoring may not be independent of their disease risk.

In a study of a dynamic population we let participants enter and leave our study at different points in time, as illustrated in Fig. 1.1.

In this population we have one person who gets the disease during follow-up (person no. 6). We have four who were under observation the entire time period of follow-up (1, 7, 9, 10). Four became members of the study group during follow-up (moved into our city) (2, 5, 8), and four left our study group during follow-up (3, 4, 5; notice that 4 even left the study twice). The *incidence rate* (IR) is defined as

(all incident cases)/(all observation time in the population at risk that gave rise to the cases)

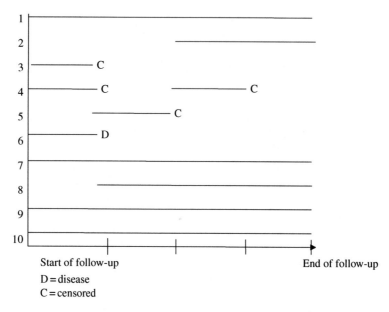

Start of follow-up   End of follow-up

D = disease

C = censored

Fig. 1.1 Ten people provide the following information during follow-up

IR, in this case, is estimated by the average rate over 2 years and it would be

$$(1)/(2 + 1 + 0.5 + 1.0 + 0.5 + 0.5 + 2 + 1.5 + 2 + 2)\text{years or } 1/13 \text{ years or } 0.077 \text{ years}^{-1}$$

Notice that incidence rates have a dimension, namely time^{-1}, in this case years^{-1}. We could of course express the same rate in months $= 1/(13 \times 12)$ months $= 0.0064$ months^{-1}, or in days, hours, or minutes for that matter. Cumulative incidence risk (or our estimate of *risk*) is an estimate of a probability with a value from 0 to 1 or 0 to 100% and has no dimension (but must be understood in the context of a given time period). We expect, for example, a smoker to have a cumulative incidence of lung cancer of about 0.10 from when he starts smoking at the age of 20 and continues smoking until he becomes 65 years of age. For a heavy smoker the CI may be close to 20%.

Calculating incidence rates requires data on the onset of the disease, which may not be known. As a surrogate the time of diagnosis is often used, or the time of the first symptoms if these are unambiguous markers of the onset of the disease, but often there are no clear early signs. When, for example, does autism begin? The first symptom may have been present very early in life, but a diagnosis cannot be made until the child has the opportunity to establish social contacts with others.

Incidence rates are measured as an average over a given time period (*incidence density*) in order to get some observations to study, although a rate is often expressed at a given point in time in common language like the speed you read from a speedometer in a car. If you drive 60 km/h it means that you drive at this speed at this moment. Only if you continue with the speed (rate) for 1 h will you travel a distance of 60 km.

Calculating Observation Time

Calculating *observation time* is a tedious job in large studies which is usually left for a computer algorithm to determine after having been provided with the appropriate dates of interest. You should, however, know what the algorithm is doing and check for a sample of data that you get the observation times you want. Take, for example, two women from a study on the use of antidepressive medication and subsequent breast cancer. Assume all events take place on January 1, and then you may have the data presented in Fig. 1.2.

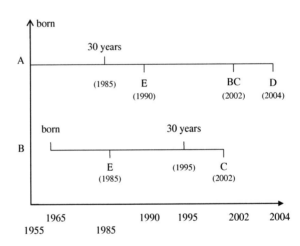

Fig. 1.2 Observation time when using antidepressants for two women. $E =$ exposure, starts medication; $BC =$ diagnosed with breast cancer; $D =$ dies; $C =$ censoring, dies in a traffic accident

These two women (A, B) will contribute 12 + 17 years to the exposed cohort. They would contribute to the exposed cohort within the age of 30–39 years with 10 + 7 years. If you consider that it would take a certain time period for an exposure (the medicine) to cause a clinically recognized cancer (BC) and if you believe that those who get breast cancer within a time period of 5 years after taking the drug therefore have a different etiology (that they are not caused by the exposure) then you would lag these results by allowing for 5 years of latency time. The observation time would then be 7 + 12 years and 7 + 7 years for all and for those within 30–39 years of age, respectively.

Prevalence, Incidence, Duration

The amount of water in a lake will be a function of the inflow of water (from rain, a river, or other sources) and the outflow (evaporation, a canal, or other types of output). The prevalence of a disease in a population will in like manner be a function of the input (incidence) of new diseased and the output (cure or death). Schematically, it will look like Fig. 1.3.

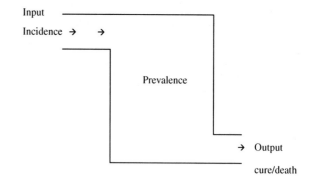

Fig. 1.3 Prevalence as a function of incidence and prevalence

In a time period where the incidence exceeds the rate of cure or death the prevalence will increase. If a cure for diabetes becomes available prevalence will decrease if incidence remains unchanged.

Under steady-state conditions the prevalence is a function of the incidence (I) and the duration of the disease (D). For a disease, such as diabetes type 1, the prevalence will increase if the incidence is increasing or if the duration of the disease is increasing. In many countries we see an increasing prevalence of diabetes and the reasons could both be an increasing incidence (inflow) or a decreasing outflow (increasing life expectancy in patients with diabetes). At least part of the increasing prevalence is due to better treatment of patients with diabetes and thus a longer life expectancy for these patients.

Under certain conditions (no change in incidence or disease duration over time, no change in the age structure) an approximate formula for the link between incidence and prevalence is

$$PP = \frac{IR \times D}{1 + IR \times D} \quad \text{or} \quad PP/(1 - PP) = IR \times D$$

PP = Prevalence proportion
IR = Incidence rate
D = Disease duration measured in the same time unit as the incidence rate

Mortality and Life Expectancy

Mortality is an incidence measure. Mortality rates are incidence rates, the number of deaths in a given population divided by the time period when we have had this population under observation. When we estimate mortality rates we try to accept that the question is not whether we die or not, but how old we become before we die. Under steady-state conditions, the incidence rate (for deaths called mortality rates (MR)) will provide an estimate of the life expectancy by taking its reciprocal values 1/MR, just like the expected disease-free time period is 1/IR under steady-state conditions in a population with no other competing causes. Since this assumption is unrealistic the reciprocal incidence rate is, rarely a good approximation to the average waiting time to the onset of the disease or the life expectancy.

Disease-specific mortality is also an incidence measure, but rather than calculating all deaths in the numerator we only calculate deaths from specific diseases. Those who die from other causes are censored; they are removed from the population at risk. Some of these censored deaths may arise from non-independent events. Dying from a stroke may, for example, share causes with death from coronary heart disease.

If we have censored observations (meaning we have competing events that end the observation before the onset of the disease itself) we often use the Kaplan–Meier method to produce a survival curve, i.e., the probabilities of dying or surviving as a function of time. Say we had a population of 10 people exposed to a deadly virus. Six of them die from the virus and one dies from other causes (censored). We would then stratify the table according to the time to the event, death, and could have the results in Table 1.1.

When it is possible to stratify on all events at the points in time where these single events happened, the probability of death is 1 divided by the population at risk at the time when a death occurs. The probability of surviving is 1 minus the probability of dying and the cumulative survival is the product of these probabilities of surviving. The probability of surviving until day 20 is the probability of surviving to day 7 × day 8 × day 9 × day 10, etc. $(1.0 \times 0.90 \times 0.89 \times 0.86 \times 0.83 \times 0.80 \times 0.75) = 0.34$.

The Kaplan–Meier survival curve will look as in Fig. 1.4.

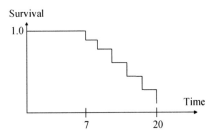

Fig. 1.4 Kaplan–Meier plot

Table 1.1 Ten people followed for 20 days

Time since exposure in days	Population at risk	Event death/censoring	Probability of death	Probability of survival	Cumulative survival Kaplan–Meier
T_i	N_i	D_i	D_i/N_i	$1 - (D_i/N_i)$	S/t
0	10	0			1.0
7	10	Death	0.10	0.90	(1×0.90)
8	9	Death	0.11	0.89	$0.80 = (1 \times 0.90 \times 0.89)$
10	8	Censoring			
11	7	Death	0.14	0.86	$0.68 = (1 \times 0.90 \times 0.89 \times 0.86)$
15	6	Death	0.17	0.83	$0.57 = (1 \times 0.90 \times 0.89 \times 0.86 \times 0.83)$
18	5	Death	0.20	0.80	$0.46 = (1 \times 0.90 \times 0.89 \times 0.86 \times 0.83 \times 0.80)$
20	4	Death	0.25	0.75	$0.34 = (1 \times 0.90 \times 0.89 \times 0.86 \times 0.83 \times 0.80 \times 0.75)$

Notice that this method of estimating risks can also be used for events other than death. If we studied patients with herpes zoster who take a new painkiller we could estimate the probability of remaining in pain over time – cumulative survival with pain. We can then calculate the probability of being relieved for the pain as a function of time in the group of patients receiving one type of treatment versus another type of treatment.

Case fatality is a cumulative incidence measure. It is the cumulative incidence (or an estimate of the probability) of dying with a disease for people who have the disease. Observation starts once the disease has been diagnosed and ends when the patient dies. Assume you have 600 new cases of monkey pox in the Congo and 30 of them die within 6 months after the start of the infection, then the case fatality is $30/600 = 0.05$ or 5%.

Life Expectancy

The usual way of calculating the *life expectancy* for a population in demography is to run a simulation study. Let 100,000 babies be born and then apply existing sex- and age-specific mortality rates to this fictitious birth cohort and see how old they will be on average when they have all died in our computer simulation. This life expectancy is therefore based on the present mortality experience and thus past exposures. It is, therefore, not a prediction (or expectancy). It is only a prediction, or expectancy, if you assume age- and sex-specific mortality will not change over time, but they have changed in the past; in fact, life expectancy has increased by 3 months every year for the past 160 years in some countries [3]. A better prediction would take changes in life expectancy over time into consideration (and other types of information as well).

References

1. Parkin DM, Whelan SL, Ferlay J, Teppo L, Thomas DB (eds.). Cancer Incidence in Five Continents, Volume VIII. IARC Scientific Publications No. 155. IARC Press, Lyon, 2002.
2. http://www.who.int/icd
3. Oeppen J, Vaupel JW. Broken limits to life expectancy. Science 2002;296(5570):1029–1031.

Chapter 2
Estimates of Associations

Incidence rates and prevalence proportions are used to describe the frequency of diseases and health events in populations. They are also used to estimate an *association* between putative determinants, exposures, and a disease. Epidemiologists often use the term *exposures* to describe a broad range of events, such as stress, exposures to air pollution or occupational factors, habits of life (such as smoking), social conditions (such as income), or static conditions (such as genetic factors). The term, exposure, is thus used to describe all possible determinants of diseases. We are interested in estimating if, and if so, how strongly these exposures are associated with a disease (increase and decrease). We do that by comparing disease frequencies in exposed and unexposed people.

In a simple situation we may observe exposed and unexposed people for a number of months (observation months), and we count newly diagnosed patients in that time. If we assume complete follow-up for 1 year and obtain the data (N = the number of people being followed up, D = disease) of Table 2.1), then one measure of association (under certain strong conditions an estimate of the effect of the exposure for the disease under study) would be the *relative risk*, RR:

$$RR = \frac{200/1,000}{100/1,000} = 2.0; \quad RR = \frac{CI_+}{CI_-}$$

The interpretation is that the estimated risk (CI, cumulative incidence) of getting the disease in the year where we had all in the population under observation (no loss to follow-up) was twice as high among the exposed as it was among the unexposed and there could be many reasons for that.

Another measure of association is the *incidence rate ratio* (IRR):

Table 2.1 Follow-up study with complete follow-up

Exposure	N	D	Observation years
+	1,000	200	900
−	1,000	100	950

J. Olsen et al., *An Introduction to Epidemiology for Health Professionals*,
Springer Series on Epidemiology and Health 1, DOI 10.1007/978-1-4419-1497-2_2,
© Springer Science+Business Media, LLC 2010

$$\text{IRR} = \frac{200/900 \text{ years}}{100/950 \text{ years}} = 2.01; \quad \text{IRR} = \frac{\text{IR}_+}{\text{IR}_-}$$

With this measure we state that the incidence rate (IR) of developing the disease per year (new cases per year of observation time among the population at risk) is 2.01 times higher for exposed than for unexposed. Note that this measure does not require complete follow-up of the cohorts.

We may also take an interest in getting an absolute measure of the difference in incidence among exposed compared with unexposed. The *risk difference* or *cumulative incidence difference* will be obtained by subtracting the two cumulative incidences $(200/1,000 - 100/1,000) = 0.10$. The rate difference will be $(200/900 \text{ years} - 100/950 \text{ years}) = 0.117 \text{ years}^{-1}$. Relative terms describe how many times the incidence rates for unexposed is to be multiplied to obtain the incidence rate among exposed. The differences provide estimates on an absolute scale. The risk is increased by 10% and the average incidence rate per year is increased by 0.117 years^{-1}.

Notice that these relative and absolute measures of association are purely descriptive. They may, under certain conditions, estimate the effect of exposure, but unless strict (and rare) conditions are fulfilled, the terminology should not promise more than is justified. We are usually interested in effects, but we measure associations. In fact, we are never able to measure effects, only to estimate them.

Usually we have incomplete follow-up even in a fixed cohort because some people leave the study for a number of reasons. They may move out of the area we have under observation (be censored), or they may die from a disease different from the one we study (be censored). Imagine a small segment of our population follow this pattern (D = the disease under study and C = censored observation). If we stop the observation at t_1, we may get the pattern seen in Fig. 2.1.

Fig. 2.1 Observation time

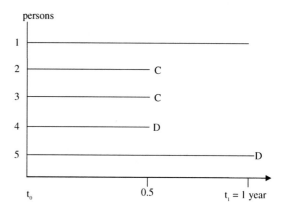

We have two diseased in our population of five people, but only two of the five were under observation for 1 year (1 and 5). An estimated CI of $2/5 = 0.40$ may be too low since 2 and 3 could become diseased after they left our study. A CI of

$2/3 = 0.66$ would be too high – we did observe 2 and 3 for 6 months and they had not been diagnosed with the disease of interest D up to that time. We can, however, use all available information by estimating the incidence rate: $2/(1 + 0.5 + 0.5 + 0.5 + 1)$ years $= 0.571$ years^{-1}.

Knowing the incidence rates makes it possible to calculate CI under certain conditions by means of the *exponential formula*

$$CI = 1 - e^{-IR \times \Delta t}$$

In this case we get $1 - e^{-0.571} = 0.435$ ($\Delta t = 1$), given the incidence rate is constant over the time period (Δt).

The risk of getting the disease over a period of 1 year is 43.5%, but this risk is subject to substantial random variation due to small numbers.

Usually, the incidence rate will not be stable over time, especially if time is age. In that case, we have to stratify the IRs over time intervals, Δ_i, where they are proximally constant, and the formula for using incidence rates to calculate risk becomes

$$CI = 1 - e^{-\Sigma_i IR_i \times \Delta_i}$$

If the disease is rare, like most cancers, the CI is close to $\Sigma_i IR_i \times \Delta_i$. The risk of getting lung cancer if you live to be 70 is approximately equal to the sum of incidence rates for the age groups 0–9, 10–19, 20–29, 30–39, 40–49, 50–59, and 60–69, multiplied by 10 for these age intervals.

For males (and females) the incidence rates of most cancers are close to 0 up to the age of 30. Let us then say the incidence rates of lung cancer for males per 100,000 observation years are: 0 (0–29), 0.1 (30–39), 0.8 (40–49), 1.2 (50–59), and 3.5 (60–69). The cumulative incidence rates up to age 70 would then be: $0.1 \times 10 + 0.8 \times 10 + 1.2 \times 10 + 3.5 \times 10$ per 100,000 years $= 56$ per 100,000 observation years, rather close to CI $= 1 - e$ $[(0.1 \times 10 + 0.8 \times 10 + 1.2 \times 10 + 3.5 \times 10)/100,000]$:

$$CI = 0.0005598 \text{ or } 55.98 \text{ per } 100,000 \text{ observation years}$$

Incidence rates and incidence rate ratios are what we normally have to measure since we rarely have the opportunity to follow a closed population over time with no censoring, and rates may often be the measure of choice.

Chapter 3
Age Standardization

When we compare disease occurrence between populations in order to estimate effects we would like to take into consideration as many factors as possible that may explain the difference except the exposure under study and its consequences. We try to approach an unachievable *counterfactual* ideal by asking the question: What would the disease occurrence have been had they not been exposed? In descriptive presentations the aim is less ambitious, but it is common practice in routine statistical tables to make comparisons that are at least age and sex adjusted.

Most diseases and causes of death vary with age and sex; thus crude incidence and mortality rates should often not be compared unless the underlying age and sex structures in the populations are similar. Age is a time clock that starts at birth and correlates with biological changes over time and cumulative environmental exposures. Therefore, most diseases are strongly age dependent. By adjusting for age by using age standardization we may, to some extent, take age difference into consideration (Table 3.1).

Table 3.1 Mortality in Greenland and Denmark. Males 1975

	Greenland			Denmark			Ratio Denmark/ Greenland
Age year	Death D_i	Observation years	Death per 1,000	Death D_i	Observation years	Death per 1,000	
<1	26	429	60.6	434	35,625	12.2	5.0
1–4	4	2,044	2.0	101	1,49,186	0.7	2.9
5–14	11	7,194	1.5	175	4,01,597	0.4	3.7
15–44	37	13,572	2.7	1,494	1,076,842	1.4	1.9
45–64	35	2,949	11.9	6,166	5,52,133	11.2	1.1
65+	47	640	73.4	19,204	2,88,834	66.5	1.1
Total	160	26,828	6.0	27,574	2,504,217	11.0	0.55

The crude overall mortality rate is seen to be higher in Denmark than in Greenland (11 and 6 per 1,000) in spite of the fact that all age-specific mortality rates are higher in Greenland (from 1.1 to 5.0 times higher). The explanation for this

J. Olsen et al., *An Introduction to Epidemiology for Health Professionals*,
Springer Series on Epidemiology and Health 1, DOI 10.1007/978-1-4419-1497-2_3,
© Springer Science+Business Media, LLC 2010

is that the population in Greenland is much younger than the population in Denmark and mortality rates increase with age: The comparison is confounded by age. The crude relative mortality rate $6/11 = 0.55$ reflects both differences in mortality rates and differences in age structure. In this case the differences in age structure and age-specific mortality rates are so large that even the direction of association is wrong. It is, however, a fact that only 6 males per 1,000 in Greenland died in 1975 while 11 per 1,000 died in Denmark. The risk of dying was higher in Denmark because the population was much older than in Greenland, not because the life expectancy was shorter in Denmark than in Greenland; in fact, life expectancy was and is longer in Denmark than in Greenland for both males and females.

The crude mortality rate is a weighted average of *age-specific mortality rates* (MR) as shown in Table 3.2. The weights (w_i) are the proportions of people within the age categories. The comparison of crude rates is age confounded because these age-specific weights differ in the two populations.

Table 3.2 Structure of the crude mortality ratio

Age year		Greenland			Denmark		
		w_i	MR	Sum	w_i	MR	Σ
<1	429/26,828	= 0.016	X 60.6	= 0.970	0.014 X	12.2	= 0.174
1–4	2,044/26,828	= 0.076	X 2.0	= 0.152	0.060 X	0.7	= 0.042
5–14	7,194/26,828	= 0.268	X 1.5	= 0.402	0.160 X	0.4	= 0.064
15–44	13,572/26,828	= 0.506	X 2.7	= 1.366	0.430 X	1.4	= 0.602
45–64	2,949/26,828	= 0.110	X 11.9	= 1.308	0.220 X	11.2	= 2.469
65+	640/26,828	= 0.024	X 73.4	= 1.751	0.115	66.5	= 7.670
Total		1.0		6.0	1.0		11.0

When we age standardize we should use the same set of age-specific weights in the comparison and we will use that as our definition of *age standardization*.

If we use an external set of weights – similar to using an age distribution in a fictitious model population – the standardization is called *direct standardization*. If we use one of the two sets of weights for the populations we want to compare we call the standardization *indirect*, although this terminology is not very informative. What is important is that data are age standardized if the age-specific mortality rates we compare are weighted by the same set of weights. There are different weights to select from and this choice should be made with care. Unless the relative mortality rates are the same in all age groups, the selection of weight will affect the result we get.

To illustrate what is done in *indirect standardization*, have a look at Table 3.3.

In this table, we take the observed number of deaths in the population of Greenland (160) and estimate how many deaths we would have expected had they had the same age-specific mortality as in Denmark. We simply take the age-specific mortality rates from Denmark and apply these to the observation time we have in each age group in Greenland ($12.2 \times 429 + 0.7 \times 2,044 + 0.4 \times 7,194 + 1.4 \times 13,572 + 11.2 \times 2,949 + 66.5 \times 640)/1,000 = 104.1$. By doing that we find an

Table 3.3 Indirect standardization using data from Table 3.1

| | Denmark | | Greenland | |
Age	Mortality rate per 1,000 observation years	Observation years	Observed number of deaths	Expected number of deaths[a]
<1 year	12.2	429	26	5.2
1–4	0.7	2,044	4	1.4
5–14	0.4	7,194	11	2.9
15–44	1.4	13,572	37	19.0
45–64	11.2	2,949	35	33.0
65+	66.5	640	47	42.6
Total	11.0	26,828	160	104.1

[a]If they had the same mortality rates as in the Danish population.

expected number of deaths of 104.1 and the standardized mortality ratio (SMR) is therefore the observed number of deaths divided by the number multiplied by 100 to produce a percent:

$$SMR = \frac{160}{104.1} \times 100 = 154$$

or, the mortality rate is on average 54% higher in Greenland than in Denmark. The weights are based on the age structure in Greenland for both the observed and the expected number of deaths, and the rates are therefore age standardized according to our definition. Notice that the SMR depends on which set of weights we use since the age-specific mortality rate ratios vary largely with age. They are especially higher in Greenland than in Denmark among the young and by selecting the population in Greenland we give more weight to the young. The SMR is an average measure given these conditions but it does not provide all the available information on mortality risks in the two populations. Important information is given in the age-specific rates. In fact, it would be misleading just to present the SMR value. It does not provide all the information we have available; the SMR is not a *sufficient statistic*.

It should also be noted that none of these comparisons take forces of selection into consideration. Since mortality is higher in Greenland, the older Greenlanders become, the more selected they will be. That is true in both populations, but more so in Greenland. For this reason we underestimate the mortality rates among the oldest in Greenland when we make comparisons with Denmark since this comparison is probably confounded by genetic factors; the oldest Greenlanders are less genetically frail than their Danish age-matched counterparts. They survived stronger forces of selection than were present in Denmark at that time.

Chapter 4
Causes of Diseases

Measures of associations remind us that diseases are not random events but results of the interplay between genes and environmental factors. We are therefore able to prevent a number of diseases, or at least to delay their time of onset by reducing the causes that are reducible. If we could convince smokers to stop smoking, provide basic health care to all, make the inactive be more physically active, reduce air pollution, eliminate the most dangerous occupational exposures, encourage people on an unhealthy diet to eat more fruit and vegetables, and make the poor more wealthy, we could prolong life substantially for many people. If we only did this by taking away exposures that people like, many would feel life was prolonged even if it was not and that is not our aim. In public health and clinical medicine we try to add life to years as well as years to life.

Although we have established a large number of disease determinants, our predictions of disease occurrence in the future are uncertain. They are like weather forecasts. They are better than predictions based on pure guesses, but they are often wrong. They are better over shorter than over longer time periods. But why are they so uncertain?

If we know the causes of a disease, why can we not be certain of their time of onset? The answers to this question are important and have been subject to much debate that is outside the scope of this book, but in short: Even if we know all causes of diseases, which we do not, we do not know if these causes will be present in the future, and even if we knew the causes there need not be a deterministic link between the cause and the effect, and that is in conflict with a common sense concept of causation. If we press the switch the light is on. Should that not happen, we would check if the power supply is functioning, if the light bulb is intact, etc. We do not believe the light failed because of chance (but chance is an explanation we frequently rely upon in epidemiology).

Our common sense concept of *causation* will tell us that given all these conditions are in place the light will be on when we press the switch. Although there is a sequence of causes, the sequence is deterministic. If the electrician we asked to repair the light said the light did not work because of bad luck we would call another electrician. In disease causation we do not have many examples of sequences of a deterministic link between the exposures and the disease. Whether there is a random element in disease causation or not is not known and may never be known because

J. Olsen et al., *An Introduction to Epidemiology for Health Professionals*,
Springer Series on Epidemiology and Health 1, DOI 10.1007/978-1-4419-1497-2_4,
© Springer Science+Business Media, LLC 2010

most diseases have many causes. What we do know is that associations appear to be probabilistic.

We would be most disappointed if the electrician we called to fix the light came up with a statement like: "if you press the switch sometimes the light is on, but sometimes it is not, and it may take years to happen and sometimes the light will be on even though nobody turned on the switch." This is, however, the kind of explanation we often have to offer in health promotion and disease prevention. We thus have to be more precise in explaining what we are talking about when we talk about disease causation because we are in conflict with commonsense concepts. Our prediction will always be uncertain because diseases have many causes and these causes may interplay in settings that may or may not be present at the time they can activate an onset of a disease. Our present understanding illustrates a substantial complexity in causation of many diseases.

Mackie elegantly illustrated how we can understand this uncertainty while maintaining our common concept of causation in his papers from the 1960s and 1970s and his landmark book from 1974 [1]. He showed how causes sometimes may activate an effect and sometimes may not, why causes appear to be probabilistic. Hume discussed causes in a global ("strong") sense as necessary and sufficient. Let us begin by explaining these global concepts.

Let E be the cause and D its effect, the disease, then the E → D path illustrates that when we have an exposure, E, we get a disease, D, and if we have D it was always preceded by E. We do not have many examples of causation in medicine that follow this pattern. The necessary part of this definition is defined by this diagram:

a necessary cause:

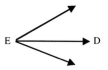

If you have the disease the cause, E, was present at some point in time before the onset of the disease, but the cause need not lead to the disease. The examples we know from the medical literature that follow this pattern usually stem from diseases where we have defined the disease to include the cause(s) (AIDS includes HIV infections in the definition, FAS (fetal alcohol syndrome) includes prenatal alcohol exposure in the definition, etc.). HIV and alcohol exposure become necessary causes according to this method of defining a disease. We have used a circular argument to make our case. That is not the same as saying we are wrong but just states that it could be wrong and we could still have generated a link that would fulfill the causal criteria. If you define a post-Christmas depression as a depression that follows 2 weeks after Christmas it does not mean Christmas is causing depression (although it could be the case). It would follow the diagram because it only illustrates a sequence of events. Depressions occur throughout the year and some will happen in the 2 weeks following Christmas due to chance alone. If we include a certain gene mutation in our definition of a given disease, then the mutation becomes a necessary "cause" of the disease whether it has anything to do with the disease or not.

A *sufficient cause* is a cause that is always followed by the disease, but the disease may have other causes as well:

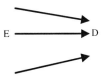

We have only few such examples, but a lack of iron or vitamin B in the diet (E) and anemia (D) could be such causes. A necessary and sufficient cause is illustrated by

$$E \rightarrow D$$

and here examples are few, if any. An exception might be single-gene disorders where the disease almost always follows the presence of the "mutation" like for PKU, cystic fibrosis, or sickle cell disease.

In fact, most of the causes we study seem to follow a pattern like this:

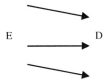

Sometimes D follows E, but not always, and sometimes D is seen for people not exposed to E.

Mackie showed that if we imagine causes acting together in concert (in what he called *causal fields*), the individual causes would follow a probabilistic pattern in populations that are characterized by the frequency of the other causes in the causal field (called component causes). At least four causes are needed to generate a pattern where none of these four causes (E_1–E_4) are necessary or sufficient in the "strong" global sense. If we imagine that we have two causal fields leading to the disease, the diagram describing the situations where none of the singular causes need to be necessary or sufficient in themselves is presented in Fig. 4.1.

E_1 (or E_3) will only lead to D in the presence of E_2 (or E_4) and the strength of the association between E_1 (and E_3) and D will depend on the frequency of E_2 (and E_4) in the population we study.

Causal field 1 (E_1, E_2) is sufficient, but not necessary (the same for causal field 2 (E_3 and E_4)). Causation follows the so-called *INUS principles*: Component causes are *i*nsufficient in themselves (require other component causes in the causal field). They are *n*ecessary within the causal field (but not in a global sense). Causal fields

Fig. 4.1 Four component
causes, two causal fields

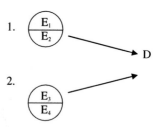

are *u*nnecessary (because there are other causal fields), but they are *s*ufficient (if they are complete).

This causal model is a useful working model in epidemiology whether it is actually true or not. Our criterion for usefulness is related to whether it fits observations and explains phenomena we observe or whether it inspires new studies. It explains, for example, that there are many different approaches in disease prevention. We may prevent D entirely if we eliminate one cause in each of the described causal fields (we need not eliminate all four). If causal field 2 accounts for 90% of the diseased, eliminating E_3 (or E_4) would reduce disease occurrence by 90% (E_1 or E_2 by 10%). There is no reason to assume that causes sum up to 100%, which follows from the fact that component causes have to operate together to produce an effect.

Very similar ideas on causation were independently developed by Kenneth Rothman and elegantly presented in his widely cited paper from 1976 (reprinted in 2004) [2].

The causal field model also explains the time lag between the onset of exposure and the disease (there is no time lag between the causal field and D, or between Hume's strong causes and their effects). The time from onset of, say, E_1 to D will be the time until the onset of E_2 (*induction time*) and the time from completion of the causal field (the start of the biological process) and until D surfaces to clinical detection (*latency time*) [2].

Causal fields will often be much more complicated than those presented here, and the causes need not operate at the same point in time or the same sequence in time. In most cases, causes probably act in complicated sequences in time. Cell modifications leading to cancer may require several steps to onset a disease, and several causes could operate during this time period. Many observations indicate that diseases should be seen in a life course perspective where different determinants (causal fields) play a role at different stages of life.

The model explains how smoking can be a cause of lung cancer, although not all smokers get lung cancer (in fact, only about 10%) and some get lung cancer without having been a smoker (about 1%). Smoking acts in combination with other causes (genetic factors, other external carcinogens) and smoking is not present in all the causal fields leading to lung cancer. We can tell the smoker that his average lifetime risk is 10% for getting lung cancer. If a smoker has a family history of lung cancer or if he is also exposed to air pollution or asbestos his risk is higher. Certain genetic factors will also put him at a higher risk, but the risk will still be far from 1.

Many smokers will live long lives and die from other causes than lung cancer. This is well in concordance with the fact that smoking causes lung cancer but only conditionally with other component causes or that the induction and latency time period may be longer than for other causes that lead to death.

It may also be of interest to note that if everyone in a population smoked 20 cigarettes per day, lung cancer might appear as a predominantly genetic disease, possibly determined by the genes that are involved in removing carcinogens in tobacco smoke from the lungs. Epidemiologists have to use variations in exposures to examine causes. If there is no variation, we have no comparable information (information on health outcomes among the unexposed). In fact, we have no one without any exposure to environmental tobacco smoke, air pollution, saturated fat, etc., at least no adult people, but we do have a variation in the levels of these exposures that allows us to compare the heavily exposed with the less exposed.

The usual pattern of disease occurrence is more like what is presented in Table 4.1.

Table 4.1 A component cause

Exposure	Disease	No disease	All
+	100	900	1,000
−	10	990	1,000

And not like in Table 4.2 (a necessary cause in the strong Hume sense).

Table 4.2 A necessary cause

Exposure	Disease	No disease
+	100	900
−	0	1,000

Nor like in Table 4.3 (a sufficient cause in the strong Hume sense).

Table 4.3 A sufficient cause

Exposure	Disease	No disease
+	1,000	0
−	10	1,000

And usually the associations between exposures and diseases are much smaller than seen in Table 4.1.

When epidemiologists talk about causes of diseases, they usually think about all the factors that increase or decrease the occurrence of diseases whether they are removable or not. Causes therefore include genetic factors as well as exposure to, e.g., a carcinogenic exposure. Philosophers may say that the cause of fire was the lighting of a match and not the presence of wood. Public health workers tend to focus on avoidable causes which would include both the removing of the wood as well as being careful with matches. If removing the wood would have prevented the fire that cause is as good as any other cause. We know that some ethnic groups have a higher incidence of prostate cancer than other ethnic groups. This is useful information in preventive medicine if it helps in identifying preventable causes of prostate cancer. There could, for example, be lifestyle factors or dietary habits that differ among ethnic groups. If it is entirely related to genetic factors we may recommend screening for prostate cancer in the ethnic group with a high risk if we have a useful screening test.

In conclusion, the component causal models explain some of the anomalies that are in conflict with common sense concepts such as (1) Why are causes not all-or-none effects? The reason is that events have more than one cause and the causal field has to be completed to onset an event. (2) Why do we see delayed effects? The delayed effects come from the time it takes from onset of the exposure until the other component causes in the causal field are in place (induction time) and the time it takes from completion of the causal field until the disease reaches a stage where it is detectable (latency time). (3) How can we understand strength of association? The strength of association depends more on the occurrence of the other component causes leading to a disease. If these other component causes are frequent in the population the strength of association is high; if they are rare the strength of association is low.

References

1. Mackie JL. The Cement of the Universe. A Study of Causation. Oxford University Press, Oxford, 1974.
2. Rothman KJ. Causes. Am J Epidemiol 2004;104(6):587–592.

Chapter 5
Descriptive Epidemiology in Public Health

Data on incidence and prevalence of diseases are needed to characterize the health of a population. Public health organizations oversee these efforts. The public health staff need to have a *community diagnosis* to set priorities. The key to this diagnosis is incidence and prevalence of diseases and the occurrence of risk factors in the population.

We need to monitor incidence data over time to identify changes in their occurrence. If the incidence is increasing and we know the causes and know how to avoid them, prevention strategies may be applied.

Comparisons of incidences between different areas have been used with great success to generate hypotheses on the etiology of diseases, and cancer rates vary, for example, largely between different geographical areas. Part of the reason for a variation could be a difference in genetic causes, but studies also show a large variation between similar ethnic groups or within an ethnic group where one part migrates from one country to another. For example, Japanese people have low incidence rates of colon cancer in Japan, but these rates increase after some time for those who move to high-risk areas, such as the USA. Rapid changes over time within the same population are usually not driven by genetic factors, although they could have a genetic component such as gene expressions depending on environmental exposures. Several observations indicate that the association between obesity and diabetes differs largely between ethnic groups, probably due to genetic factors that are activated under certain lifestyle conditions.

Table 5.1 shows *direct age standardized* incidence rates (in this case standardized by applying the study rate to a common set of age-specific weights (world population)) and incidences of the cancers. Some of these cancers show large variations, e.g., for prostate cancer. Other cancers have much less geographical variation, e.g., leukemia.

Descriptive data are also used to demonstrate social differences in diseases and mortality. In the UK, e.g., occupational mortality tables have been produced for more than a century. From the offices of Population Census and Surveys causes of death are displayed according to occupational and social groups [2].

Table 5.2 shows cumulative incidence of symptoms of food poisoning 24 h after having eaten the indicated food items. Due to tradition, these cumulative incidence

J. Olsen et al., *An Introduction to Epidemiology for Health Professionals*,
Springer Series on Epidemiology and Health 1, DOI 10.1007/978-1-4419-1497-2_5,
© Springer Science+Business Media, LLC 2010

Table 5.1 Rates standardized to world population,[a] per 1,00,000 per annum [1]

Population	Stomach Male	Lung Male	Leukemia Male	Prostate Male	All sites Male	Breast Female	Cervix uteri Female	Female
Cali, Colombia	57.5	17.5	5.2	23.2	(25.25)	27.3	75.6	(25.75)
Alameda county	24.4	43.8	8.3	65.3	(26.51)	38.6	30.5	(18.78)
Birmingham, UK	25.2	73.3	5.3	18.4	(26.00)	51.1	13.6	(19.50)
Japan, Miyagi prefecture	95.3	15.6	4.4	3.2	(21.51)	11.0	20.6	(15.04)

[a]Rates taken from *Cancer Incidence in Five Continents*, Vol. II.

Table 5.2 Differences in food-specific attack rates in an outbreak of food-borne illness [3]

	Persons who ate specified food				Persons who did not eat specified food				Difference in attack rates
	Ill	Well	Total	Attack rate (%)	Ill	Well	Total	Attack rate (%)	
Shrimp salad	8	4	12	67	15	21	36	42	+25
Olives	19	13	32	59	5	13	18	28	+31
Fried chicken	10	33	43	23	4	2	6	67	−44
Barbecued chicken	17	1	18	94	3	27	30	10	+84
Baked beans	12	13	25	48	12	10	22	55	−7
Potato salad	17	20	37	46	8	6	14	57	−11
Macaroni salad	9	15	24	38	15	10	25	60	−22
Root beer	23	23	46	50	0	2	2	0	+50
Bread	8	9	17	47	18	13	31	58	−11
Neapolitan cream pie	1	2	3	33	21	21	42	50	−17

proportions (risks) are called *attack rates* and differences in attack rates are used to generate hypotheses of specific food items that should be further investigated (in this case, for example, barbecued chicken).

The World Health Organization has produced papers on the *global burden of diseases* to remind us of how unequally health is distributed in the world and how closely many of our health indicators correlate with poverty [4] (Fig. 5.1).

The public health worker needs to be familiar with more measures of disease occurrence and the relation between these measures. Often, they will have to work with secondary data that only approximate the information needed to make exact calculations. They should know when these approximations are good enough for the purpose at hand and when they are not.

In public health it is furthermore often useful to estimate the proportion of the diseased that could be avoided if we eliminate the exposure, the *attributable fraction*. If the exposure is a "strong" necessary cause for the disease the calculation is simple since there will be no cases if we eliminate the exposure. We have no cases

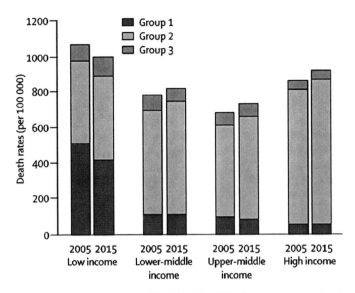

Fig. 5.1 Projected crude death rates per 100,000 by World Bank income groups for all ages, 2005 and 2015 [5]

of smallpox because the smallpox virus has been eradicated, at least outside a few laboratories. In most other instances, the situation is more complicated. Assume we have a fixed cohort like in Table 5.3.

Table 5.3 Obesity and fetal death

Obesity	N	Fetal deaths	RR
Yes	1,000	20	
No	2,000	20	2.00

We could then ask ourselves how many of the 20 fetal deaths could be avoided had the pregnant women not been obese. Unfortunately, we have no way of knowing that. They were obese and cannot be both obese and not obese in the same pregnancy. That is why the argument is contrary to facts – contrafactual (we cannot roll back the film and let them go through the same pregnancy without their obesity). We can, however, imagine or predict what would have occurred if they had not been obese.

What we can do is to assume that the non-obese provide an estimate of what would be the risk for the obese had they not been obese – that is a very strong assumption and most likely wrong to some extent. Given we make that assumption we calculate that $20/2,000 \times 1,000 = 10$ fetal deaths would be expected among the obese had they not been obese. The attributable fraction among exposed would be that 10 out of 20 cases could be prevented $((20 - 10)/20 = 0.50$ or 50%. If we spell out how we calculated that number, it becomes

$$\frac{(CI_+ - CI_-)1,000}{CI_+ \times 1,000} = \frac{CI_+ - CI_-}{CI_+}$$

and if you divide by the CI_- you get

$$\frac{RR - 1}{RR}$$

CI = cumulative incidence; RR = relative risk.

The attributable fraction in the entire population would be $10/40 = 0.25$ or 25%; that can be calculated as

$$\frac{\text{All exposed cases}(RR - 1/RR)}{\text{All cases}} = \frac{20(RR - 1/RR)}{40} = 0.25$$

In this population, we estimate that it would be possible to prevent 25% (10 out of 40) of all fetal deaths if we could get all obese to become normal weighted. Notice that the attributable fraction in the population depends on the RR and the exposure distribution in the population.

These calculations are meaningless and misleading unless we are confident that the associations are causal. There could be a common etiology to obesity and fetal death or there could be bias or other types of confounding that were not controlled in the analysis. Attributable fractions are not measures to be used unless there is strong evidence from many sources pointing toward causal links between the exposure and the outcome. Obesity and fetal death is not yet a good candidate for calculating "attributable fractions," although it has been done. We need to know much more about this association before it becomes a candidate for this particular type of measure.

In some textbooks you find the term *etiologic fraction* to mean the same as "attributable fraction." Some use the term etiologic fraction to mean the fraction of people that had the disease because of the exposure. We need a causal concept to understand the meaning of such a term. In our component causal model all component causes in a causal field are necessary causes within this field, but we can define the last component cause (if it is known), the one that onsets the disease, as the cause of interest for the etiologic fraction. Notice that if the causal field consists of stationary genetic factors and an external toxic exposure that onsets the disease, we can emphasize this cause as we did when we said the fire was not caused by the presence of wood but by the lighting of a match.

In this understanding, the etiologic fractions need not be of the same magnitude as the attributable fraction. One can also imagine that the attributable fraction is 0 and the etiologic fraction is greater than 0. Assume an aggressive smoking cessation program that works for some smokers but makes other smokers continue smoking although they were prepared to quit the habit. If both groups are of equal size the attributable fraction of the smoking cessation program could be 0 and the etiologic fraction is represented by those who quit smoking because of the program. Notice, however, that it makes little sense to talk about *the* cause of a disease when several component causes are in the field leading to the disease. They are all necessary causes in that causal field.

Graphical Models of Causal Links

Over the years epidemiologists have used graphical presentations of the exposures, confounders, and diseases they study. More formal rules for depicting these diagrams have been presented [6] and especially the *directed acyclic graphs* (DAGs) play an increasingly important role in setting up the strategy for selecting variables to be collected and for selecting the appropriate way to analyze data. The causal links in the DAG are directed by arrows. It is acyclic since no directed paths form a closed loop. Not all causes need to be in a DAG, but if two or more variables share the same cause then this "parent" of the two variables should be in the DAG. A much simplified DAG on the link between air pollution and asthma could look like this [6]:

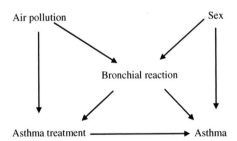

This diagram indicates that there is a direct link between treatment and asthma. There are two alternative paths (back-door paths) from air pollution to asthma via bronchial reaction, or via bronchial reaction and sex. These back-door paths need to be controlled. We furthermore notice that if we control bronchial reaction we open another back-door path via air pollution to sex and asthma. We call bronchial reaction a collider in the path between air pollution and sex. Since both arrows point toward bronchial reaction we would establish a link between air pollution and sex since they are both causes of this bronchial reaction. A collider can therefore lead to a misleading result if it is included improperly in the analysis. The DAG tells us we should not just include all potential confounders in our analysis.

A simpler description of a collider could be presented by the below diagram.

We would expect no link between candidate genes for asthma and socioeconomic status since genes are allocated in a randomized way at conception according

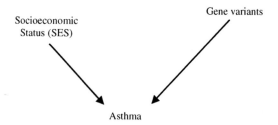

to Mendel's laws. Among children with asthma you would expect an association between these genetic factors and SES according to this diagram. Good social conditions may lead to asthma as well as certain genetic factors; therefore these two variables become associated in children with asthma (and to a lesser extent in children without asthma).

An intermediate factor is in the causal pathway from the exposure to the end point under study and should not be controlled in the analysis.

The causal links between a high fat diet and coronary heart diseases (CHD) could be like this:

$$\text{High fat diet} \rightarrow \text{high se-cholesterol} \rightarrow \text{CHD}$$

Including se-cholesterol would eliminate the caused association we take an interest in. If the association is like this:

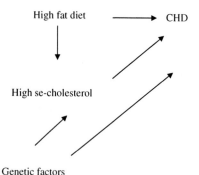

including se-cholesterol would open a back-door path from diet to genetic factors and CHD that cannot be controlled unless the genetic factors are measured and included in the model. Se-cholesterol is a collider between diet and genetic factors. Had there been no link from genetic factors to CHD, controlling for se-cholesterol would estimate the unbroken link from diet to CHD.

DAGs have been a useful tool to clarify and communicate ideas and hypothesis. It is a tool to make predictions that can be tested and the diagram shows you how to analyze your data. It is useful not only when a strategy for confounder adjustment is discussed, but also for identifying selection and information bias. The drawback is that DAGs become very complicated in many real-life situations because the causal structure is often complicated. Many variables are often measured by proxies (or instrumental) variables. We may be interested in the cumulative exposure to specific components of air pollution, but we may only have general data on the air quality in the area where people live, for example. The use of instrumental variables adds to the complexity of the DAG just as including forces of selection that keep eligible people out of the study tends to make DAG difficult to interpret.

For more information on DAG the reader is referred to Chapter 12 in Rothman et al. (2008) [7].

References

1. Muir Calum, et al (eds.). Cancer Incidence in Five Continents, Volume V. IARC, Lyon, 1987.
2. Occupational Health Decennial Supplement. Office for National Statistics (ONS) & Health and Safety Executive (HSE), published every ten years, ISBN=9780116916181.
3. Last JM, Wallace RB (eds.). Maxcy-Rosenau-Last. Public Health & Preventive Medicine, 13th Edition. Appleton & Lange, Norwalk, Connecticut/San Mateo, CA, 1992.
4. Lopez AD, Mathers CD, Ezzati M, Jamison DT, Murray CJL (eds.). Global Burden of Disease and Risk Factors. Oxford University Press/The World Bank, New York/Washington, DC, 2006.
5. Strong K, Mathers C, Leeder S, Beaglehole R. Preventing chronic diseases: how many lives can we save? Lancet 2005;366(9496):1578–1582.
6. Greenland S, Pearl J, Robins JM. Causal diagrams for epidemiologic research. Epidemiology 1999;10:37–48.
7. Rothman KJ, Greenland S, Lash TL. Modern Epidemiology, 3rd Edition. Lippincott, Williams and Wilkins, Philadelphia, 2008.

Chapter 6
Descriptive Epidemiology in Genetic Epidemiology

Occurrence Data in Genetic Epidemiology

Genetics has come to play an increasingly important role in studies of health and disease driven both by new technologies that enable these studies (chromosome analysis, DNA sequencing, genotyping) and by our recognition of the key role of genes and genetic variation in disease causation. Humans have 23 pairs of *chromosomes* made up of some 3 billion *nucleotides* (A, C, G, and T) of DNA. There are over 20,000 *genes* scattered across the human chromosomes, most containing in their DNA sequences the information for the amino acid sequence and time/place of expression of a particular protein. We receive one chromosome (and one copy of each of the genes on that chromosome) from our mother and one from our father. Variation in the DNA sequence can result in different *alleles* or forms of the gene and these individual differences are inherited according to *Mendel's laws* of transmission resulting in dominant, recessive, or X-linked forms of inheritance. This variation in the *DNA* sequence is found about once in every 1,000 nucleotides and as of this writing more than 5 million of these variants are well characterized. The variation occurs in two common forms. The most common and studied are *SNPs* or single nucleotide polymorphisms – changes in a single DNA nucleotide at a single position (A for G, for example) that are easy to characterize and enumerate. Since we have two copies of each chromosome, one from each parent (and each gene on those chromosomes), we can define a genotype as the type of each of the two possible variants we might have (AA, AG, or GG for an A/G containing SNP). Technology allows the assay of anywhere from one to one million of these per person very cost effectively. The second common form of variation is CNVs or *copy number variants* where long segments of DNA may be present in zero to many copies. When these segments include genes they can result in the absence of a gene product (if both parents contribute zero copies) to a many-fold increase above the average amount of gene product if multiple gene copies are present. CNVs, while clearly of great biological importance, present more challenges in analysis and are less well characterized than SNPs as of this writing and so we will use SNPs in most examples to follow.

Many traits – from health outcomes to behavior and wealth – have a tendency to run in families. Families share not only environmental factors (including social

J. Olsen et al., *An Introduction to Epidemiology for Health Professionals*,
Springer Series on Epidemiology and Health 1, DOI 10.1007/978-1-4419-1497-2_6,
© Springer Science+Business Media, LLC 2010

factors), but also genetic factors. Epidemiologists have traditionally looked for environmental causes for variations in health outcomes, while geneticists have focused on genetic factors of importance for health. The interaction between these two research traditions has been surprisingly slow in emerging (the International Genetic Epidemiology Society was founded in 1991), although many researchers in both areas agree that the determinants of most health outcomes are to be found in the interaction between genes and environment. Not only are both genes and environment etiological factors (component causes in the causal fields), but, in addition, the effect of an environmental factor often depends on the genetic background on which it acts, and vice versa.

Genetic factors play a central role in a broad range of *monogenic diseases* (i.e., diseases caused by mutation in one gene and inherited by Mendel's laws) from cystic fibrosis to Huntington's disease and early-onset dementia. Most common diseases (as well as most common traits like height or eye color), however, are not monogenic, but are more likely to be influenced by a large number of environmental and genetic factors and their interactions. The technical development and dramatic decline in cost have allowed genetic analyses on a minimal amount of biological material, e.g., millions of genotypes (the genetic constitutions of the individual) can be generated from a saliva sample or a dry spot of blood. This has been instrumental in being able to incorporate genetic information into large-scale epidemiological studies.

In genetic epidemiology it is studied if, how, and why some health outcomes cluster in families, so some central questions are as follows:

- Does the trait or disease under study cluster in families?
- Are there combinations of diseases that cluster in families?
- If so, what is the relative influence of genetic and environmental factors?
- What are the specific genetic variants and environmental factors influencing the trait or disease?
- How do the environmental and genetic factors interact?

In answering these questions genetic epidemiology encounters challenges known from both epidemiology and genetics like heterogeneity in clinical presentation and etiology: The same disease can have a broad clinical spectrum, and the same clinical features can have very different etiologies. As in other epidemiological studies it is critical that there are well-defined criteria for the disease or trait under study. Furthermore, if possible, *genotyping* should be done without knowledge of the disease and *phenotyping* without information on genotypes (blinding) because both the genotyping and the phenotyping come with some measurement errors.

Clustering of Traits and Diseases in Families

There are a number of obstacles in determining the degree of familial clustering of a disease, in particular for diseases with manifestation late in life (e.g., dementia). Many family members will be too young to be at risk of having the disease, whereas others die before the typical time of diagnosis. Furthermore, in studies where the participant needs to return a questionnaire and participate in interviews about family occurrence, there is a risk that families with several affected members are more likely to participate or be detected because these families may be particularly interested in studies of familial clustering of this disease. Studies of conditions or diseases which are diagnosed early in life, and for which population-based reliable register information exists, are less vulnerable to such biases, although they are subject to Berkson's bias (p. 131) if you study associations between diseases in the same person. Clusters also occur by chance, and diseases will cluster in some families due to chance alone. The key occurrence measure of familial clustering is the recurrence rate for different degrees of relatives to the index case, i.e., the case that brings the family into the study. As indicated in Fig. 6.1 such recurrence risks will be compared with the overall population frequency in the population from which the cases were ascertained.

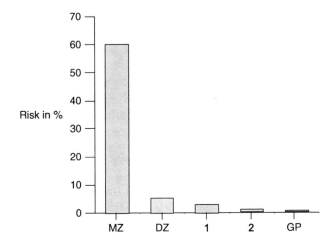

Fig. 6.1 Recurrence risk for relatives of an index case with cleft lip and palate [1]

The risk for the relatives is given for "zero"-degree relatives, i.e., the co-twin to a monozygotic twin (MZ) with cleft lip and palate, and similarly for first-degree relatives (sibs including dizygotic twins (DZ), parents, and children), second-degree relatives (grandparents, uncles, nieces, half-sibs), and third-degree relatives (e.g., cousins). GP indicates the risk in the general population. The risk for a first-degree relative (4%) is 40 times the risk for a random person in the general population (0.1%).

The recurrence risk is of interest in the clinical setting where questions are asked such as: "I have a brother with cleft lip and palate. What is the risk that my child will have the disease?" This kind of question is classic in traditional genetic counseling for monogenic diseases but also of importance for multifactorial diseases which cluster in families. The recurrence risk pattern can also provide information about the effect of genes: whether they act additively or multiplicatively, and how big an effect a single gene is expected to have.

The Occurrence of Genetic Diseases

Genetic disease can be used to describe a broad range of disorders from those caused by chromosome abnormalities or single-gene disruptions to complex multifactorial conditions resulting from the interplay of multiple genes and environmental factors. Single-gene disorders have a long history in public health and genetic epidemiology. *Phenylketonuria (PKU)* was described by Ivar Asbjørn Følling in the 1930s [2] as a recessive biochemical disorder of amino acid metabolism that, untreated, leads to profound mental retardation. *Robert Guthrie* [3, 4] developed a cheap and efficient test for PKU that, coupled with the recognition that an early dietary limitation of phenylalanine in the diet could prevent the disease manifestations, led to the first effective population-based newborn screening tests. The PKU model is now widely applied throughout the developed world for a wide range of biochemical disorders as well as hypothyroidism and hemoglobinopathies. One hemoglobin disorder, sickle cell anemia, was first described as a molecular disease by *Linus Pauling* in 1949 [5], and in the 1950s it was recognized that carriers for this autosomal recessive disease were resistant to *falciparum* Malaria while the affected homozygotes had a high mortality in early childhood. A third common recessive disorder, cystic fibrosis (CF) was one of the first human disorders to have its gene identified using genome mapping technologies, and the evolution of these technologies is now enabling the application of genetic testing as one additional method available to the epidemiologist and clinician in evaluating the role of genetic factors in disease etiology.

Another public health success has been the near elimination of the health consequences of Rhesus blood group (Rh) incompatibility between mother and fetus. An Rh+ fetus carried by an Rh− mother can induce an antibody response which results in the destruction of fetal red blood cells and subsequent anemia which, when severe, can result in death. Recognition of this genetic incompatibility led to *prenatal screening* and treatment of affected infants as well as effective prevention through the use of antiglobulins given to the mother during and following pregnancy to prevent the induction of the antibody response which would be exacerbated in future pregnancies.

Prenatal testing also achieved prominence on a population scale when amniocentesis allowed collection of fetal cells for evaluation of chromosome anomalies such as Trisomy 21 (Down's syndrome). Currently such prenatal screening also includes ultrasound evaluation of fetal organs and maternal serum testing to determine risks for chromosomal aneuploidy and neural tube defects. In the aggregate these testing options allow a better descriptive epidemiology and introduced new screening tools.

Single-gene and chromosomal disorders are now easy to define and describe with high degrees of reliability. They are not limited to the pediatric age groups. Adult onset disorders such as the autosomal dominant cardiomyopathies or long QT syndrome have also been defined and testing has been made available. Current major challenges are now focused on those more common yet complex disorders that have an underlying genetic component but where cause may involve multiple genes as well as environmental triggers that make the identification of specific risk components difficult. Disorders such as type 2 diabetes, inflammatory bowel disease, cardiovascular disease, obesity, dementia, and others are all common, yet complex, making genetic risk factor identification both more compelling and more challenging. The role of the *apolipoprotein E (ApoE) gene*, and in particular the E4 allele, in predisposing to Alzheimer's disease, was until a few years ago one of the few successful factor identifications to date for a common disease of adult onset. But recent successes in finding genetic risk factors for age-related macular degeneration, type 2 diabetes, breast cancer, and myocardial infarction suggest that genomic tools enable elucidation of population-based genetic risk factors. It is critical for the student to be aware of the ongoing developments in these areas in order to be able to provide more effective care to patients and also to facilitate involvement of patients in appropriate studies aimed at increasing knowledge and improving treatment. It is an area with a rapid development of technology that stretches statistical techniques to their limit.

Common diseases can also arise as part of the expression of single-gene Mendelian conditions or as a complex trait as defined above. The clinician or public health specialist needs to acknowledge the differences in mechanisms and implications for families as well as population planning. If stroke, myocardial infarction, hypertension, cancer, or diabetes, for example, arise as part of a dominant disorder their frequency may be much higher in an extended family than would be predicted by the prevalence of that disorder. This uneven distribution will have implications for presymptomatic screening in an at-risk family and for recognizing it as a source of etiologic heterogeneity which will need to be incorporated into public health planning. In developed countries most deaths are due to cardiovascular diseases and cancer (about one half of all deaths from these two) with accidents, diabetes, Alzheimer's, and suicide making up other significant categories. Each of these, excepting accidents, have well-recognized genetic components whose categorization and understanding will contribute to designing better methods of prevention and treatment.

References

1. Christensen K. The 20th century Danish facial cleft population – epidemiological and genetic-epidemiological studies. Cleft Palate-Craniofac J 1999;36:96–104.
2. Følling A. Über Ausscheidung von Phenylbrenztraubensäure in den Harn als Stoffwechselanomalie in Verbindung mit Imbezillität. Hoppe-Seyler's Zeitschrift fuer Physiologische Chemie 1934;227:169–176.
3. Lesser AJ. Phenulketonuria and the Guthrie test. Pediatrics 1963;32:940.
4. Guthrie R, Susi A. A simple phenylalanine method for detecting phenylketonuria in large populations of newborn infants. Pediatrics 1963;32:338–343.
5. Pauling I, Itano HA et al. Sickle cell anemia a molecular disease. Science 1949;110(2865): 543–548.

Chapter 7
Descriptive Epidemiology in Clinical Epidemiology

We live in the era of *evidence-based medicine* where "true believers" tend to disregard anything but randomized clinical trials (RCTs) even when assessing the impact of any intervention or diagnostic procedure. However, there are several shortcomings in RCTs, for instance the ability to assess long-term effects and rare outcomes. (Randomized trials are described in Chapter 9.)

Descriptive epidemiology can sometimes be used in order to assess to what extent an intervention has had an impact, especially with regard to long-term effects and outcomes. However, such an approach is not without problems, and caution should be used when minor changes in estimate of associations are used to infer causality. For instance, a slight decrease in prostate cancer mortality in some populations during the twenty-first century, notably in the USA, has been used to "sell" the message that *prostate-specific antigen* (*PSA*) screening and/or new therapeutic strategies have had beneficial effects. The existence of slow growing prostate cancers that will produce no or only mild clinical symptoms within a natural life span, combined with differences over time in diagnostic intensity, as well as changes in the way of reporting underlying causes of death, can at least partly explain such trends. Prostate cancer is probably the most unsuitable of all cancer forms to assess the impact of new interventions based on changes in incidence. This becomes evident if one compares temporal trends in incidence and mortality in prostate cancer between Sweden and Norway, two populations with very similar ethnic roots and lifestyles. There is a 50% higher incidence of prostate cancer as well as prostate cancer mortality in Sweden than in Norway [1].

This probably mirrors differences in the diagnostic intensity with regard to the incidence but may also affect cause-specific mortality figures. It is hard to tell the difference between dying from prostate cancer and dying with prostate cancer.

There are good uses of descriptive epidemiological data to evaluate an intervention. The following three different examples illustrate that – one dealing with recommendations given to the general public, the second with screening, and the third changes in the treatment over time.

J. Olsen et al., *An Introduction to Epidemiology for Health Professionals*,
Springer Series on Epidemiology and Health 1, DOI 10.1007/978-1-4419-1497-2_7,
© Springer Science+Business Media, LLC 2010

Sudden Infant Death Syndrome (SIDS)

SIDS is defined as the sudden unexpected death of an infant aged younger than 1 year where the circumstances of death have failed to provide a sufficient alternative explanation. Most SIDS deaths happen within the first 8 months of life, usually around 3–4 months. Until the 1990s young mothers, male sex, preterm and/or low birth weight infants, and maternal smoking had been identified as risk factors for SIDS and the incidence was around 2–3 per 1,000 live births. A study during the late 1980S and early 1990s from New Zealand demonstrated that sleeping in a supine position was an independent risk factor which subsequently led to recommendations worldwide to parents to let their children sleep on their backs, as illustrated by, for instance, the "Back to Sleep" campaign in the UK in 1991. The incidence of SIDS then declined dramatically during the next few years (Fig. 7.1).

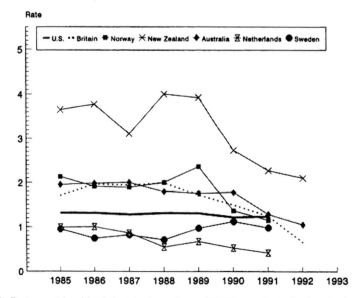

Fig. 7.1 Postneonatal sudden infant death syndrome (SIDS) rates in the USA and selected other countries, 1985–1992 [2]. These rates are calculated as the number of SIDS deaths, <27 days and <1 year of age per 1,000 live births. The 1992 SIDS rates are provisional

This drop in incidence with a 75% reduction in many different populations occurring about the same time following these new recommendations indicates a causal link, especially as changes in smoking habits, frequency of preterm deliveries, and diagnostic procedures had not changed more than marginally during this relatively short time period.

Cytological Screening for Cervix Cancer

Cancer of the cervix is one of the most common cancers in women, especially in developing countries, and is a major cause of premature death in middle-aged and older women. The introduction of Pap smear screening in the late 1960s was done in order to reduce morbidity and mortality of cervical cancer. Screening will lead to detection and removal of pre-malignant (cancer in situ) lesions with a simple surgical procedure, thus reducing both incidence and mortality of this cancer. Descriptive epidemiological data were used to evaluate these programs. Data from Sweden, for instance, show a drop in the incidence of squamous cell cancer of the cervix starting in the late 1960s followed by a drop in the mortality in cervix cancer 5 years later but an increase in the incidence of cancer in situ (Fig. 7.2).

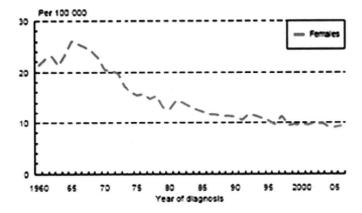

Fig. 7.2 Incidence of cancer of the cervix (ICD–7:171) [3]

These findings support a beneficial effect of this program. However, there have been other changes which could explain these trends, such as changes in smoking habits, sexual education, better access to health care. To further assess the screening program the incidence data can be modeled taking into account both birth cohort and time period effects (effects related to what happened during the time of birth or in the calendar time of follow-up). Since the screening procedure, in Sweden as in other countries, was primarily aimed at younger women when it was introduced in the late 1960s, we would expect to see a decrease in birth cohorts that were offered screening which is seen in Fig. 7.3.

The drop in incidence of cervix cancer following the introduction of the screening is related to a decrease in incidence in the younger birth cohorts starting in the 1930s and 1940s.

Fig. 7.3 Change in incidence
for cervical cancer according
to age in different time period
[4]

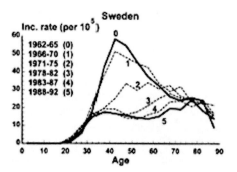

Changes in Treatment of Juvenile Diabetes

Insulin treatment in *juvenile diabetes* was introduced in the late 1920s and diabetes
nephropathy emerged as a long-term complication for these patients. Close to 50%
suffer from nephropathy 20 years after starting the treatment. In the late 1960s substantial changes in the treatment of juvenile diabetes were introduced. Until then
a standard insulin regimen consisting of a single morning dose with a long-acting
insulin was the norm, sometimes combined with a short-acting insulin. In the 1970s
a more aggressive therapy became the norm with multiple doses, which increased

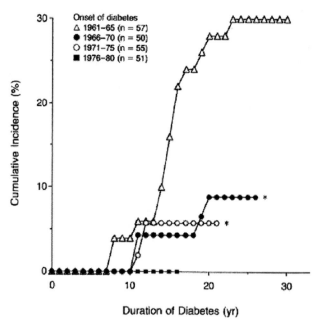

Fig. 7.4 Cumulative incidence of persistent albuminuria in patients with diabetes according to
duration of diabetes and calendar time of diagnosing [5]

further in the 1980s. During the same period educational programs as well as means for self-monitoring were added but would these new strategies have an impact on the long-term adverse outcomes in juvenile diabetes patients?

In a study consisting of only 213 patients in a defined area in Sweden all individuals with juvenile diabetes diagnosed before the age of 15 were identified from 1961 to 1980. Through the patient records the investigators were able to assess the existence of persistent albuminuria, a pre-stage nephropathy, in all patients (Fig. 7.4).

Figure 7.4 shows a substantial improvement over time indicating that aggressive treatments possibly combined with more self-care decreased persistent albuminuria.

These three examples serve to illustrate that in selected instances well-conducted descriptive epidemiological studies can be used to evaluate new interventions, especially long-term effects and the occurrence of rare events such as SIDS.

References

1. Kvåle R, Auvinen A, Adami HO, Klint A, Hernes E, Møller B, Pukkala E, Storm HH, Tryggvadottir L, Tretli S, Wahlqvist R, Weiderpass E, Bray F. Interpreting trends in prostate cancer incidence and mortality in the five Nordic countries. J Natl Cancer Inst 2007;99(24):1881–1887.
2. Willinger M, Hoffman HJ, Hartford RB. Infant sleep position and risk for sudden infant death syndrome: report of meeting held January 13 and 14, 1994, National Institutes of Health, Bethesda, MD. Pediatrics 1994;93(5):814–819.
3. http://www.socialstyrelsen.se/Lists/Artikelkatalog/Attachments/9325/2007-42-16_20074216. pdf
4. Gustafsson L, Pontén J, Zack M, Adami HO. International incidence rates of invasive cervical cancer after introduction of cytological screening. Cancer Causes Control 1997 Sep;8(5): 755–763.
5. Bojestig M, Arnqvist HJ, Hermansson G, Karlberg BE, Ludvigsson J. Declining incidence of nephropathy in insulin-dependent diabetes mellitus. N Engl J Med 1994;330(1):15–18. Erratum in: N Engl J Med 1994 Feb 24;330(8):584.

Part II
Analytical Epidemiology

Chapter 8
Design Options

Common Designs Used to Estimate Associations

Epidemiologists use population experience to learn about associations between environmental factors, lifestyles, food intake, treatments, poverty, genes, etc., and diseases. We do that by observing and analyzing what people do to themselves or what is being done to them related to the health problems they have. To be a student of the occurrence of diseases as a function of different exposures is to be a student of epidemiology. Since cause–effect relations unfold over time, both in terms of age and calendar time, time plays a crucial role in these analyses and disease occurrence is best studied from the start of exposures and in the time to follow, especially for exposures that change over time, as it can be done in a follow-up study. To obtain information on this population experience a more cost-effective strategy can sometimes be applied by sampling cases (rather than exposed and unexposed) and so-called controls. This is just another way of harvesting the underlying population experience as will be demonstrated later. Sometimes it may be possible for the epidemiologist to set the conditions for exposure allocation. If we set the conditions for the exposure in order to learn about the health effects of these exposures, we are using an experimental design by definition, often with the intention of avoiding some of the sources of bias that threaten many observational designs. The randomized controlled trial is the most frequently used experimental epidemiologic design. Within these broad groups there are many variants. Most of these designs are outside the scope of this short introductory text.

To think about causal effects, epidemiologists often use counterfactual reasoning. Women who use hormonal drugs to treat menopausal problems have a given occurrence of, e.g., cardiovascular diseases, but what would the occurrence have been had they not taken the hormones? That is of course not observable since nobody can be using and not be using hormones at the same time, but it is possible to imagine that these women had not used the hormones. To estimate what the occurrence would have been had they not taken the hormones, we unfortunately have to use a different group of women who did not use the hormones under study. We select these women in the hope that they will provide the expected disease occurrence for the exposed, had they not been exposed. Whether we succeed or not in providing a valid

J. Olsen et al., *An Introduction to Epidemiology for Health Professionals*,
Springer Series on Epidemiology and Health 1, DOI 10.1007/978-1-4419-1497-2_8,
© Springer Science+Business Media, LLC 2010

comparison group we do not and cannot know for sure. Therefore, we should not speak lightly about causal effects but use the term associations to describe the contrast between disease occurrence for exposed and unexposed. If we say an exposure is associated with a disease, it means just that – nothing more, nothing less; a given exposure level has a disease occurrence that differs from what we see at another exposure level, in a particular data source, and that can be so for many reasons.

When we have to decide between different design options, we cannot always select the design we expect will provide the best possible counterfactual contrast. Such a design would often be the randomized controlled trial, but conducting a trial may be out of the question for ethical reasons, or it may be impractical, too costly, or take a long time to conduct. To evaluate the possible effect of a given screening test on long-term mortality may take decades and the screening test may be outdated when results are available. For ethical reasons we cannot design an experimental study to see if a given drug is fetotoxic in pregnant women, not even among women who have already decided to terminate their pregnancy. Over time some women will, however, use new drugs by accident or by choice, and we can and should try to make the best possible use of the information they provide.

Many more aspects have to be taken into consideration when planning a study than the quality of the designs, but if we compromise too much on quality we may be better off without the study. In the long run, a collection of many low-quality studies may cost more research money and do harm if the results are wrong. A single, large randomized trial may be cost-effective if it is ethical and possible to do. Side effects related to taking post-menopause hormones (HRT, hormonal replacement therapy) is an area where a randomized trial was long overdue when it was finally done [1].

Taking limited time and funding into consideration, the discussion on study design selection (from inexpensive to expensive) could go like this, using a study on cell phones and brain cancer as an example.

Ecological Study

If we had national (or regional) data on mobile phone use and brain cancer, we could quickly produce an *ecological study* comparing frequencies of mobile phone use or number of mobile phones in use per 1,000 people and brain cancer incidence for populations. We may plot these data with a time lag of 5 years because we believe there will be some time lag between the exposure and disease onset. If an association exists, we might find data like those plotted in Fig. 8.1.

Although such a graph may look convincing there are several considerations to make: The graph is not based on individual level data and therefore does not relate cancers to individual mobile phone users. We do not know if it is the mobile phone users that develop cancer (*the ecological fallacy*). There are many other factors that correlate with mobile phone use in the populations and maybe the association is caused by these factors (confounders). Better diagnostic tools may be able to pick up cancers that were previously undetected or detected at a later stage. These better

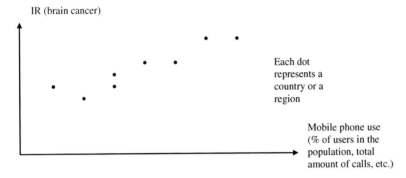

Fig. 8.1 Ecological study on mobile phone use and cancer incidence rates (IR)

diagnostic facilities may well correlate in time with mobile phone use since they both depend on the economic and technological developments.

We could conduct a cross-sectional study, *a survey*, or use data from an existing large ongoing survey with data on mobile phone use and brain cancer at a given point in time (the time of data collection). The simplest display of such a survey is summarized in Table 8.1.

Table 8.1 A cross-sectional study

Mobile phone users	Brain cancer	No brain cancer	All
Yes	a	b	N_1
No	c	d	N_0

The prevalence ratio is

$$PR = \frac{a/N_1}{c/N_0}$$

Such a survey needs to be very large to provide a reasonable number of prevalent cases of brain cancer, and this design is a more obvious choice when both the exposure and the disease are more frequent. If we have the data and PR shows an association (PR>1) our concerns will be as follows:

1. We do not know the causal direction. Perhaps brain cancer leads to mobile phone use because patients need to be in contact with their social network. Or the opposite may be more likely. Brain cancer patients may isolate themselves or prefer a more personal contact than what can be achieved over the phone. The first situation would produce a positive association, the latter a negative association and both would be spurious and non-causal for the hypothesis of interest.
2. The causes of brain cancer may correlate with mobile phone use. We could take these factors into account in the analyses if we knew them, but in this case we do not.

3. The reporting of mobile phone use may be in error (wrong or inaccurate) and perhaps more so for brain cancer patients, although they only report present use of the phones in a cross-sectional study. If mobile phone use has been a widely suggested cause of brain cancer, brain cancer patients may over-report their mobile phone use in the search for an explanation of the cancer. Further, we compare recall from a sick brain with recall from a "normal" brain. In any case, present use is only of interest if it correlates well with past use (during a possible etiologic window). The exposure data we have are not from the right time period.
4. Not all those invited will participate in surveys. If, e.g., brain cancer patients are less likely to participate it will not in itself distort the PR, but if brain cancer cases who are not mobile phone users more often decline to take part in the study than brain cancer patients who use mobile phones, an elevated PR could be a result of this selection bias. Similar selection bias could occur among the non-brain cancer patients but then it would tend to mask an association.

Case–Control Study

The next design in line to consider could be a *case–control study*. We select all cases of brain cancer in the population under study and a sample (controls) from the population that gave rise to the cases. We now record their phone use from the time period in which we think the carcinogenic process was activated. The simplest data lay-out would look like Table 8.2 (as in the survey, but the recording is now longitudinal – we try to obtain exposure data at the time period in which we believe the carcinogenic process took place, for example 5–10 years before the onset of cancer).

Table 8.2 A case–control study

Exposure history	Cases	Controls
Yes	a	b
No	c	d

$$[OR = \frac{a/c}{b/d}]$$

Depending on how controls were selected, this odds ratio (OR) could estimate the incidence rate ratio (IRR) for brain cancer among mobile phone users compared to non-users. If this estimate is greater than 1 it would indicate an association between mobile phone use and brain cancer, but

1. Are the recalls of phone use back in time accurate and comparable for cases and controls? One would think that brain cancer may interfere with cognitive functions and thus with recall of past phone use. If cancer patients over-report phone use in the past (perhaps they are more sensitive to having had something close to the brain), this could explain the observation. This source of bias is a serious problem, especially when the hypothesis is well known by the responders.
2. Selection bias could explain the association if exposed cases are more likely than unexposed cases to accept an invitation to take part in the study, and that could easily happen if the purpose of the study is revealed at the time of recruitment. Although it is not possible to give exact guidelines on an acceptable proportion of non-responders, if but more than 30% refuse to participate selection bias is of major concern. Selection bias could, however, play a role even if the proportion of non-responders is much lower, and there may be no selection bias even if many more refuse to take part in the study.
3. And, as before, other potential causes of brain cancer may correlate with phone use.
4. Further, a large source population is needed to provide a sufficient sample size to detect a small association.

Cohort Study

Next in line would be the most straightforward design, the *cohort study*. Select heavy phone users and people who do not use mobile phones and follow them over time (years or even decades). The simplest display of such a study is presented in Table 8.3.

Table 8.3 A cohort study

Exposed	Disease	Observation time
Yes	a	t_1
No	c	t_0

$$[IRR = \frac{a/t_1}{c/t_0}]$$

If such a study shows an IRR above 1 it would speak in favor of a causal association, but

1. Causes of brain cancer could correlate with mobile phone use and cause a spurious association (confounding).
2. Some of the exposure and disease data may be in error, but if brain cancer diagnosing is made without taking phone use into consideration and phone use is

registered before the onset of brain cancer this type of error would often lead toward an attenuation of the IRR. And it should be possible to obtain a large exposure contrast in countries where only part of the population uses mobile phones.

3. Although non-participation is less of a problem in the follow-up study since participants take part without knowing whether they will be brain cancer patients or not, the selection may cause other problems. Older people may, for example, be more likely to refuse taking part in the study, reducing the number of cancer events. If only one sex or ethnic group accepts the invitation we will have no way of knowing if our results will apply to the people we did not recruit to the study.

4. Change of habits and phone type over time complicates the analysis, especially if we do not know which types of exposure to check for. Furthermore, there are other sources of radio frequency exposures in the population, although not many with such a direct exposure to the brain.

The drawback is that you have to wait for years, perhaps decades, to get an answer. And the study has to be large with many thousands of exposed and unexposed depending on the expected effect.

Experimental Study

If we imagine we could obtain permission and compliance to implement an *experimental design* where we decide who will be phone users and who will not (or who will perhaps exclusively use hands-free phones that would not expose the brain and hand-held sets), we would flip a coin to let heads or tails decide whether the person will be a phone user, or a non-user (in practice we will let a computer "flip a coin" or use another method of randomization). The display of such a study, in its simplest form, could be as in Table 8.4.

Table 8.4 A randomized trial

Exposure	Disease	Observation time
Yes	a	t_+
No	c	t_0

$$[IRR = \frac{a/t_+}{c/t_0}]$$

Should this IRR be high, it would speak quite strongly in favor of a causal association if all participants used mobile phones according to the protocol, but results could still be due to chance or shortcomings in the design such as incomplete follow-up. In general, this type of design is less bias prone than other designs if compliance to phone use is kept according to the protocol, but the design is often expensive because the study needs to be large with a long follow-up time, and it is often not feasible in practice, as in this case.

In the discussed example, the ecological design will be important since even a small increased risk in phone use will produce many new cases because the exposure is very frequent. If such a frequent exposure does not correlate with brain cancer incidences in the population, the exposure is probably not a strong cause of the disease.

In practice, non-experimental designs are important for making new "discoveries," to identify new risk factors of diseases. Experimental designs are usually reserved to evaluate established hypotheses or to evaluate new medicines before they are released on the market. Both observational and experimental designs are "epidemiologic designs." Some people have the misconception that epidemiology only covers non-experimental designs, but the discipline is not defined by its methods but by its subject of research.

The most important designs will be described in greater detail in the following.

Reference

1. Cuzick J. Is hormone replacement therapy safe for breast cancer patients? Editorial. JNCI 2001;93(10):733.

Chapter 9
Follow-Up Studies

The Non-experimental Follow-Up (Cohort) Study

If you want to study determinants (exposures) of the transition from healthy to diseased or death, or from diseased to non-diseased, you have to record the sequence of causes, treatments, and end points in time; you need to have longitudinal recordings in most situations. If the exposure is obesity and the outcome is type 2 diabetes, you need at least one recording of obesity in time. Obesity is defined as a body mass index (BMI) of over 30 (a man with a weight of 95 kg and a height of 1.75 m will have a BMI of $95/1.75^2 = 31.0$ and thus be obese).

Having identified a certain number of obese individuals (e.g., males, 40–49 years of age), you then follow these people for the next, say, 10 years and record the number of new cases of type 2 diabetes in the cohort. Epidemiologists use the term *cohort* for a group of people who are followed over time (a cohort was originally a term used in the Roman army for a subset of a legion). Say 10% develop diabetes during the period of follow-up, the cumulative incidence (if 100 out of 1,000 obese had type 2 diabetes) would then be $100/1,000 = 0.10$ or 10%. Although this figure is useful, it does not tell us whether obesity is a risk indicator of type 2 diabetes or not. To obtain that information, you need to know what the expected cumulative incidence would be had the obese not been obese. That information is not available.

In the absence of this information, we select a group of non-obese men who we believe have the same risk of diabetes as the obese would have had if they had not been obese. We would at least make sure that we select unexposed with the same age structure and follow them over the same time period and calculate their cumulative incidence. The more precisely we are able to formulate our hypothesis, the better we are able to select exposed and unexposed for the study. In the simplest version of a cohort study, the data would look like what is displayed in Table 9.1.

Given these data we may then calculate the relative risk as

$$RR = (100/1,000)/(50/1,000) = 2.00$$

J. Olsen et al., *An Introduction to Epidemiology for Health Professionals*, Springer Series on Epidemiology and Health 1, DOI 10.1007/978-1-4419-1497-2_9, © Springer Science+Business Media, LLC 2010

Table 9.1 Type 2 diabetes in the obese and non-obese cohorts

Obesity	N	Disease	Observation years
+	1,000	100	9,500
–	1,000	50	9,750

and the incidence rate ratio (IRR) as

$$IRR = (100/9{,}500 \text{ obs. years})/(50/9{,}750 \text{ obs. years}) = 2.05$$

A relative risk may be high because the numerator is higher than the denominator or because the denominator is much smaller than the numerator and this may be seen as a trivial fact, but the point of departure (the numerator or the denominator) may make a difference. If obesity is doubling a high disease risk, it may be more serious from a public health point of view than if it was doubling a low risk of, say, type 1 diabetes. Type 2 diabetes is much more frequent than type 1 diabetes in most countries, and type 1 diabetes is usually a more serious disease than type 2 diabetes. A doubling of the risk of type 2 diabetes would in our example mean an 18% increase in absolute risk and a 0.2% increase of type 1 diabetes if the risk for non-obese is 0.1% over the follow-up time period.

In order to provide information that illustrates actual risks, we may calculate absolute measures of differences in risks and rates. The risk differences (RD) for type 2 diabetes given in Table 9.1 would be

$$RD = (100/1{,}000) - (50/1{,}000) = 0.05$$

and the incidence rate difference (IRD)

$$IRD = (100/9{,}500 \text{ obs. years}) - (50/9{,}750 \text{ obs. years}) = 0.054 \text{ years}^{-1}$$

Studying Risk as a Function of BMI

This obesity example is a bit too simple for several reasons. Although there is an arbitrarily defined cut-off level for obesity, there is another limit for being overweight and one for being underweight. If we think of our study as a study of fixed cohorts we would probably like to include at least three cohorts in the study: obese, overweight, and normal weight. We would then add at least one line to Table 9.1. The new table could look like Table 9.2.

Using the same comparison group – those with a normal weight – we show that the association may follow a *dose–response pattern*, and in a large sample we could even describe type 2 diabetes risk as a function of much finer BMI strata. If this

Table 9.2 The risk of diabetes in obese, overweight, and normal weight cohorts

BMI	Weight	N	Disease	RR	RR
30 or greater	Obese	1,000	100	2.0	1.33
25–29.9	Overweight	1,000	75	1.5	1 (reference)
18.5–24.9	Normal	1,000	50	1.0 (reference)	0.667

association is linear, we have a constant RD across each BMI unit; the cumulative incidence increases with a constant RD for each unit change of BMI (Fig. 9.1).

Fig. 9.1 Cumulative incidence (CI) for diabetes and BMI

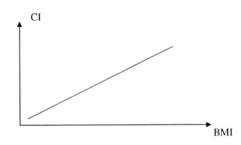

Table 9.2 would follow such a structure because the risk difference is constant from strata to strata (0.025).

If the RR increases with a constant value across each BMI level, the association is exponential and would look like Fig. 9.2.

Fig. 9.2 Cumulative incidence (CI) for diabetes at BMI

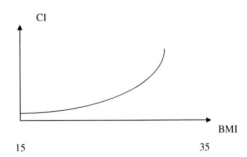

Figure 9.2 illustrates a constant RR from one strata to the other. In Table 9.2 the RR from normal to overweight is 1.5, but from obese to overweight it is $(100/1,000)/(75/1,000) = 1.33$. Had we had 112.5 diseased among the obese, the RR from overweight to obese would also be $1.5 = (112.5/1,000)/(75/1,000)$ and the dose–response curve would be exponential. Figure 9.2 illustrates an exponential curve with an RR of 2 for each step of 5 BMI units.

If we change to logarithms of the CIs the graph between BMI and CI would again be linear. CI increases with a fixed log RR value for each BMI level.

The log plot would look like Fig. 9.3.

Fig. 9.3 Diabetes and BMI

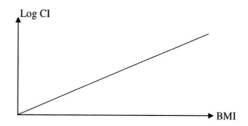

Longitudinal Exposure Data

In our cohort design we measured BMI at a given point in time at which we also start counting follow-up time regardless of the fact that their obesity or being overweight may have started a long time ago. We identified a population at risk (free of diabetes at baseline) and counted observation time from the starting time. To capture changes in BMI we would need repeated (longitudinal) measures of BMI over time along with data on the onset of type 2 diabetes. We would then have to work on incidence rates where we calculate observation time as time being in a certain weight category. Assume Fig. 9.4 describes one man's BMI over time.

Fig. 9.4 BMI in one person
over a time period of 10 years

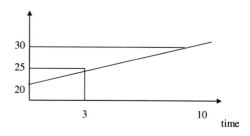

This person would contribute 3 years of observation time within the normal BMI group (BMI < 25), 7 years within the overweight group (BMI 25–29), and none within the obese group (BMI ≥ 30) since he only reaches this level at the end of observation time. We would have to repeat these BMI measurements over time for all members of the cohort to calculate incidence rates within these BMI groups. If the person displayed in Fig. 9.4 got type 2 diabetes after 7 years of follow-up time, he would contribute to the incidence rate with 1/7 years in the overweight group and 0/3 in the normal weight group, and these measures we have to add up for everybody in the study. The data we get would look like what you see in Table 9.3.

This would be an appropriate way to analyze the data in lack of a specific hypothesis on the association between BMI and type 2 diabetes. If we had reason to expect that there is a time lag between becoming obese and type 2 diabetes or between a given change in weight and the disease, the calculations would be more complicated. In fact, there could be numerous different ways of analyzing the data,

Table 9.3 Incidence rates and relative incidence rates as a function of weight status

Weight	Observation time	Diseased	IRR
Obese	t_{++}	D_{++}	$(D_{++}/t_{++})/(D_0/t_0)$
Overweight	t_{+}	D_{+}	$(D_{+}/t_{+})/(D_0/t_0)$
Normal weight	t_0	D_0	1.0 reference

and we may need rather complicated statistical techniques to perform some of the analyses.

We also need technical skills to make the groups comparable on characteristics that may play a role for the risk of type 2 diabetes. Sex, age, a family history of diabetes, diet, and physical exercise correlate with diabetes risk, and we may need to adjust for these factors in order to come closer to estimating unconfounded associations.

When we say the aim is to select unexposed with the same disease risk as exposed had they not been exposed, we take into consideration that we do know something about other risk factors that should be controlled in the analysis. Our comparisons will not just rely on simple tabulations as those presented previously. Our comparisons may, for example, be made within strata defined by other risk factors. A stratum of such a table could look like Table 9.4.

Table 9.4 Stratified analysis

Family history	Sex	Age	Obesity	Observation time	Disease
0	M	30–39	Yes	t_i+	D_i+
			No	t_i-	D_i-

Within this *stratum* we compare disease occurrence among obese and non-obese and sum up associations from all strata to make a combined estimate or that is how data were analyzed back in time. Now *stratified analyses* are unfortunately too often replaced with statistical modeling.

Different Types of Cohort or Follow-Up Studies

At baseline, at the start of follow-up, we may be able to classify people as exposed or unexposed. An accidental toxic exposure of short duration may leave people in a local area exposed or unexposed. From this given point in calendar time we follow up all subjects in our exposed and unexposed cohort. This we will call a fixed cohort. More often the situation will be that we start our study at a given point in calendar time and recruit eligible candidates into the study over time and move them to the

Fig. 9.5 Observation time
according to exposure

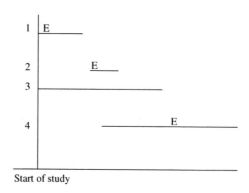

Start of study

exposed cohort when they become exposed, for example when they start taking a new type of medicine or move into an area with heavy air pollution (Fig. 9.5).

Eligible candidates enter our cohort at different time periods. When they become exposed we move them to the exposed cohort and start counting observation time from the time of exposure (or later if we want to take into consideration a latency time period). Person no. 4 will thus start accumulating observation time in the unexposed cohort (when he enters the cohort) and then change to the exposed cohort during follow-up. In this cohort we have a dynamic recruitment to the exposed cohort during follow-up; it is a cohort with open entry. It could be a cohort of patients with diabetes where we may be interested in a specific new treatment as the exposure. Since exposures may cause diseases long after exposure has stopped we do not always remove people from the exposed cohort when exposure stops. If we did a study on car accidents and mobile phone use we would, however, remove people from the exposed cohort when they stopped using mobile phones while driving. We have no reason to believe that a history of mobile phone use in itself affects the risk of car accidents. Such a study would have both an open entry and an open exit.

We could also have a situation as depicted in Fig. 9.6.

Fig. 9.6 Observation time
according to exposure (E)

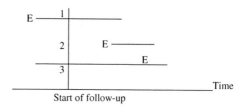

Start of follow-up

We would start counting observation time from the start of follow-up for persons numbered 1 and 3 but not from the time of exposure (for no. 1). The reason is that we have no complete surveillance of all possible eligible candidates for the study before we set up our follow-up surveillance program. Person number 1 is a candidate for the study because he did not leave the region or die before the start of follow-up.

Some call this time from start of exposure to start of follow-up *immortal observation time* because they can only enter the study if they are alive at the start of follow-up. In like manner, we start calculating observation at age 60 if we are interested in mortality rates from 60 years of age. If we take an interest in lung cancer risk for people who have smoked at least 40 years, we start calculating observation time when they have accumulated this number of exposed years.

Should we be able to identify all eligible candidates from a point dating back in time and all end points (diseases) of interest during follow-up we may reconstruct observation time back in time. We call such a study *a historical cohort*. This design is often used in occupational epidemiology where it may be possible to identify all factory workers in a given plant back in time, for example based upon employment or union records.

The terms cohort study and *follow-up study* are often used to describe the same type of design although some would stress that in a cohort the aim is to follow all until they get the disease in question, die from other causes, or reach the date that terminates the study. Following cancer incidence in a given region by setting up a cancer registry and counting the dynamically changing population of those who remain within the region is therefore not a cohort study. It is a follow-up study for that region if we have the entire population under surveillance, but there is no intention of tracking people who leave the region.

The main design feature for a follow-up or cohort study is to select exposed and unexposed and follow disease occurrence in these groups over time. If the diseases we take an interest in are rare or have a long induction and latency time we may not have the time to wait for a result or the funding needed to establish a large follow-up study. The case–control study then becomes an attractive alternative given certain conditions are fulfilled.

Chapter 10
Case–Control Studies

A follow-up study on chronic diseases usually needs to be large with a long follow-up period to provide a sufficient number of cases to be informative. Most of the participants in the study will provide little information since they will remain disease-free. A case—control sampling strategy may sometimes be possible and it can usually be conducted at a much lower cost than a follow-up.

We should keep in mind that we are still harvesting the same population experience of disease occurrence among exposed and unexposed. This population experience is our only source of information. We are using the changing exposures in the population over time to learn about exposure–disease associations. We only consider a more economic approach to obtaining the information we seek. To demonstrate the basic sampling principles, we start with the follow-up study and examine how we calculate relative measures of associations. Assume that we have the data in Table 10.1 from a fixed cohort study with no loss to follow-up (all are followed from the start of follow-up and until the observation period ends, or until the onset of the disease under study).

Table 10.1 Follow-up study

Obesity	N	Disease	Observation time
Yes	N_1	D_1	t_1
No	N_0	D_0	t_0

The following measures can be estimated based on the data given in Table 10.1:

$$\text{RR(relative risk)} = \frac{D_1/N_1}{D_0/N_0} \text{ which can also be written as OR} = \frac{D_1/D_0}{N_1/N_0} \quad (10.1)$$

$$\text{IRR(incidence rate ratio)} = \frac{D_1/t_1}{D_0/t_0} \text{ which can also be written as OR} = \frac{D_1/D_0}{t_1/t_0} \quad (10.2)$$

$$\text{OR(odds radio)} = \frac{D_1/(N_1 - D_1)}{D_0/(N_0 - D_0)} \text{ which can also be witten as OR} = \frac{D_1/D_0}{(N_1 - D_1)/(N_0 - D_0)} \quad (10.3)$$

J. Olsen et al., *An Introduction to Epidemiology for Health Professionals*,
Springer Series on Epidemiology and Health 1, DOI 10.1007/978-1-4419-1497-2_10,
© Springer Science+Business Media, LLC 2010

If we have no loss to follow-up we can estimate the relative risks as the ratio between the cumulative risks for exposed divided by the cumulative risk for the unexposed. The incidence rate ratio is in like manner based on the two incidence rates, and the odds ratio reflects the odds for disease occurrence among the exposed divided by the disease odds among the unexposed. Notice that OR can also be expressed as the exposure odds among diseased and the exposure odds at baseline in the entire cohort (10.1) or the odds of exposure time during follow-up (OR) or the exposure odds among non-diseased (the right-hand side of equation 10.2). The OR (disease odds ratio) in the cohort study is seen to be similar to the exposure odds ratio among cases and non-cases (10.3).

The rearranged right side of the equations illustrates that if we have a disease register and the possibility to classify the exposure data retrospectively, we may produce the same relative measures of association by selecting all cases (the right-side numerators) and a sample of the denominators (right-side denominators). To estimate relative risks we need controls to estimate the ratio of exposed and unexposed at baseline (N_1/N_0). To estimate IRR we need controls to estimate the ratio of exposed and unexposed observation time (t_1/t_0) and to estimate OR we need controls to estimate the proportion of exposed and unexposed non-diseased at the end of follow-up ($(N_1-D_1)/(N_0-D_0)$).

Assume that a follow-up study provides the results summarized in Table 10.2.

Table 10.2 Follow-up study with observation time

Obesity	N	Disease	Observation time
Yes	10,000	200	9,900 years
No	30,000	300	29,850 years

Then we obtain

$$RR = \frac{200/10,000}{300/30,000} = 2.00 \tag{10.4}$$

$$IRR = \frac{200/9,900}{300/29,850} = 2.01 \tag{10.5}$$

$$OR = \frac{200/9,800}{300/29,700} = 2.02 \tag{10.6}$$

With access to a disease register for this population we may be able to identify all cases in the population and by interviewing or by using stored biomarkers or existing records to classify the diseased as exposed or unexposed in the proper time period when the exposure may cause the disease. With the same set of cases and three different sets of controls we can estimate RR, IRR, and OR.

We call the first type of a case–control study the *case–cohort study*. We select all cases at the end of follow-up. Then we select a random sample of everybody in the cohort at the start of follow-up, at baseline. The size of the control sample can be larger or smaller than the case set, but usually we select a sample of a similar size as the number of cases, or we take 2–5 times more controls than cases. If we can afford five times as many controls as we have cases we will in most situations obtain almost all the available information from the underlying source population and still record exposure data for much fewer people than if we had done a follow-up study.

The size of the sample determines the statistical precision we achieve and in many situations where the disease is rare, we will select all the cases we can get that fulfill our diagnostic criteria. If costs of getting information from cases and controls prohibit us from selecting more controls than cases, then a 1:1 design (an equal number of cases and controls) is usually the best choice.

Case–Cohort Sampling

Assume we select one control per case and we have no sampling variation, the study would produce results as in Table 10.3.

Table 10.3 Case–cohort sampling

Exposure	Cases	Controls
Yes	200	125 (10,000/40,000 × 500)
No	300	375 (30,000/40,000 × 500)
All	500	500

$$OR = \frac{200/300}{125/375} = 2.00$$

Our OR estimates the risk ratio or relative risk if we sample from the entire cohort at baseline independently of their later disease occurrence (the case–cohort sampling). Note that controls will include cases with the same frequency as the cumulative incidence indicates.

Density Sampling of Controls

In order to estimate the IRR, we design a *case–control study with density sampling*. The cases are the same, but controls now have to estimate the distribution of exposed and unexposed observation time in the underlying cohort as seen from the right-side denominator in Table 10.1. If we do not take sampling variation into consideration we get the results in Table 10.4.

Table 10.4 Case–control study with density sampling of controls

Exposure	Case	Controls
Yes	200	$124.5 = (9{,}900/39{,}750 \times 500)$
No	300	$375.5 = (29{,}850/39{,}750 \times 500)$
All	500	500

$$OR = \frac{200/300}{124.5/375.5} = 2.01$$

One way to obtain an estimate of the exposed/unexposed observation time is to select controls at the onset of case identification. Among all in the underlying cohort at risk of getting the disease we select controls at random at the point in time when a case is diagnosed. Thus, observation time among those at risk, whether they are exposed or unexposed, determines the probability of being sampled. This sampling procedure allows controls to become cases if, after having been selected as controls, they get the disease under study. A person may also be sampled more than once as a control since the probability of selection is only determined by the duration of the observation time. We will estimate IRR by calculating the odds ratio (OR) in Table 10.1. This method will also work in case–control studies performed in populations that are based on a dynamic cohort if we, for example, want to study the association between a genetic marker and childhood diabetes. We may select patients with newly diagnosed diabetes in our study region and among disease-free children at the time of diagnosis of the cases and we select controls, but this particular study will be rather robust to design modifications. For example we could sample controls at different time slots equally distributed over the time period of case ascertainment. Whether we allow controls to be recruited to the case group if they get the diagnosis under study or not is also a minor issue in this study, because childhood diabetes is a rare disease. Deviations from the ideal design become more critical if we study an exposure that changes over time, like infections or air pollution, or if we study a frequent disease like spontaneous abortions early in pregnancy. The principles of density sampling are illustrated in the population of 10 people coming in and out of our study area during the time of case–control recruitment (Fig. 10.1).

C indicates the point in time where a participant leaves our study area, dies from other causes, or is no longer under observation (censored). D indicates onset of the disease under study. When person number 7 gets the disease, persons numbered 1, 2, 3, 4, and 10 belong to the population at risk and are candidates for being sampled to the control set. When person number 3 becomes a case, persons numbered 1, 4, 5, 8, and 10 are candidates for being sampled to the control set. If person number 3 was selected as a control for case number 7 we will keep this person in the study as both a control and a case. Since cases leave the population at risk they cannot be selected as controls from that time.

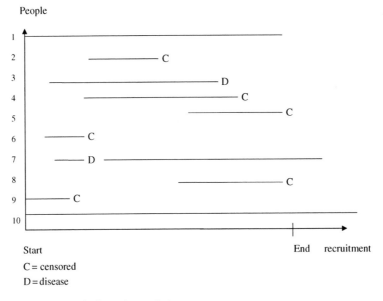

People

Start   End   recruitment

C = censored
D = disease

Fig. 10.1 Follow-up of a dynamic population

Case–Non-case Study

The third type of a case–control study we will call a *case–non-case study*. First, we select all the cases. Then we sample a set of controls from the non-cases at the end of follow-up. Without taking sampling variation into consideration, we end up with the data as in Table 10.5 (sampling based on data in Table 10.2).

Table 10.5 A case–non-case study

Exposure	Cases	Controls
Yes	200	124.1 = (9,800/39,500 × 500)
No	300	375.9 = (29,700/39,500 × 500)
All	500	500

$$OR = \frac{200/300}{124.1/375.9} = 2.02$$

The *exposure odds ratio* equals the *disease odds ratio*, and odds are close to proportions (P) when the proportions (P) are small (Odds = $P/(1 - P)$). From this it follows that the disease OR is close to the RR if the disease is rare among both exposed and unexposed (as in our example). You will find this described as *the rare disease assumption* in many textbooks. The two other case–control designs need no rare disease assumptions as long as it is accepted that people may be selected more than once to the study.

The case–non-case design was inspired by Stuart Mill's methods of agreement and disagreement in search for causes or events [1]; we try to identify causes by looking for similarities in exposures among cases and by trying to find what separates exposures among cases from exposures among non-cases. Furthermore, the design leads to a simple statistical analysis since we have no overlap of cases and controls. The design does not take into consideration that being disease-free is a question of time and can lead to misleading results. Imagine, for example, that you study a pregnancy biomarker that changes over gestational time. If you want to see if this biomarker is a risk factor for preterm birth you have to select controls at the same gestational week, not women who gave birth at term (non-cases). If the biomarker changes with gestational time, there will be a difference between cases and non-cases, even when the biomarker does not predict preterm births.

The case–control design described in this section assumes it is possible to identify members of the population that gave rise to the cases and sample from them. We also assume that we have a disease register that captures everyone with the disease in a given time period.

It is not always possible to identify the population at risk within some geographical boundaries at given points in time. In many countries it is hardly ever possible. We may have a hospital that receives all patients with a serious disease (say, type 1 diabetes) from a given catchment area. We may know the geographical borders of this catchment area, but we may not have a list of all the people living in this area at a given point in time that could serve as our sampling frame. If it is out of the question to make a complete population registry for the entire population, we may produce a small local population registry, for example by identifying all people living within a short distance of the case person, and sample at random among these people. We call these controls *neighborhood controls*. We may also use the case person's area phone number to define the "neighborhood" and at random (*random digit dialing*) select a phone number within this area code that belongs to a person and use him/her as a control. These methods may not work if we are studying exposure related to the close neighborhood, like air pollution and socioeconomic standards. The random digit dialing methods may be biased when having a phone, being reachable on the phone, or having a number of phones correlate with the exposures we study.

Patient Controls

In many case–control studies, other patients (patients with another disease than the disease under study) are used as controls. That works well if the exposure distribution among these *patient controls* is interchangeable with the exposure distribution among proper controls (randomly sampled from the population that gave rise to the cases). The problem is that we do not know if this is the case, and it is probably seldom fully so. It is not so if the exposures under study cause or prevent the "control" disease. Use of other disease groups may even be biased if exposure is not causally related to the control diseases but when the exposure under study correlates with the probability of being diagnosed or hospitalized. If so, the exposure distribution will not reflect the exposure distribution in the source population that gave rise to the cases. Assume we take an interest in smoking as the exposure and use colon cancer controls. If coffee drinking protects against colon cancer, as some studies suggest, colon cancer patients may have a lower smoking prevalence than what is present in the population that gave rise to our cases (proper controls should estimate that prevalence). Since smoking and coffee habits often correlate we would overestimate the risk unless we adjust for coffee intake in the analyses. Assume we want to study if a specific infection in childhood causes type 1 diabetes and we use children coming into the hospital with fractures as controls. If we want to study a cause–effect association with short duration, this will not work. Infections tend to keep children less active and may therefore prevent against accidents and injuries. Children with asthma may not be appropriate either since infections may initiate or worsen an asthma attack. But the design may be appropriate if we believe the infection causes type 1 diabetes with a delay of months or years. Use of patient controls may be a useful option (and perhaps the only option) in many situations.

It may be very difficult to find a disease that for certain is neither caused nor prevented by the exposure under study if the exposure interferes with several disease mechanisms, such as infections or obesity. Studying the effect of a single gene may be simpler, although a common gene variant like ApoE-4 is known to be associated with several diseases (e.g., cardiovascular diseases and Alzheimer's disease).

There are many variations over these basic case–control designs. They all aim at harvesting the underlying population experience in order to estimate the association between exposures and the disease. The most used design is the case–control study with some type of density sampling since we rarely have the luxury of having a well-defined cohort to sample from at baseline. If we do have such a cohort we will often use a case–cohort design, especially if you have valuable biological material from the entire cohort and you intend to use this cohort to study several outcomes. A random sample from this cohort at baseline may then be used as a common set of controls for several case series. Density sampling produces one specific set of controls for each case series. There is, however, one caveat when sampling controls at baseline.

If the time between sampling of the biological material and the occurrence of the disease under study is not short, a slight modification is needed. Within this fixed cohort sample you will not only sample among those that were at risk when the cases were diagnosed. You will also sample people who were censored before cases surfaced to clinical detection and you have to take that into consideration when analyzing the data since not all were under observation for the same amount of time due to censoring. Analyzing data using survival techniques may solve the problem.

Secondary Identification of the Source Population

Under ideal conditions we have a disease register that captures everybody with the disease in a given population and we are able to sample controls from this source population and all participants in our study. These conditions are seldom if ever completely fulfilled. Not all with the disease are diagnosed or at least not diagnosed at the same stage of the disease. If we want to use a case–control design to estimate the effect of a newly introduced screening test the results will most likely be misleading. The aim of the screening test is usually to diagnose a disease at an earlier stage, to bring prevalent but yet undetected patients to our attention. Until steady-state conditions are reached, a case–control study may show screening as a risk factor of the disease just because it moves the diagnosing forward in time.

Assume we want to study whether a given food item causes diarrhea among tourists in Thailand. We may have to restrict our study to severe cases of diarrhea that always (or almost always) come to medical attention, but we will have no way of identifying all tourists in Thailand at the time of data collection. Members of the source population have to be defined by the case series as people who would become cases if they had the disease that brought the cases to medical attention. Clearly that is not a simple definition to use since not only the severity of the disease plays a role, but also access to health care from a practical and financial point of view. Designing case–control studies under these conditions requires much experience [2] and should be left to professional epidemiologists.

In short, the main design feature in a case–control study is the selection of cases and a random sample from the population that gave rise to the cases. The aim is to reconstruct the data we need to estimate the relative effect measures in the underlying population. When this is done we estimate if the exposed have the same disease risk as the unexposed, not if the exposure is more frequent among cases than among controls. We are not comparing cases and controls but exposed and unexposed.

Case–Control Studies Using Prevalent Cases

In the described case–control designs the aim has been to provide data on factors associated with the transmission from healthy to diseased. The aim is to identify incident cases and reconstruct their exposure history before the onset of the disease within the time period we believe to have causal importance. Sometimes prevalent cases are recruited to a case–control study because recruitment of new cases may take too long. If you want to study the determinants of multiple sclerosis (MS), you would need a very large source population to obtain a sufficient number of incident cases within a reasonable time period because the incidence rate in the population is low. Since you have MS from when you are diagnosed until you die, the prevalent pool of MS patients will be 20–40 times larger than the annual incidence, depending upon the life expectancy of MS patients. Using prevalent cases of MS may therefore provide the sample size you would need, but bigger is not always better and it comes with a price to use prevalent cases as explained in the following.

Assume you had access to a large prevalent pool of cases from a large health survey, perhaps including records of patients with diabetes. You may want to study whether a specific genetic polymorphism is associated with diabetes, and if this genetic testing is expensive you might not be able to perform the test on everyone in the survey. You may select all with diabetes and then take a random sample from all in the survey to serve as your controls. Blood samples could then be collected and analyzed from cases and controls. The simplest display will be as presented in Table 10.6.

Table 10.6 A case–control study with prevalent cases of diabetes

Genetic mutation	Cases	Controls
Yes	a	b
No	c	d

$$OR = \frac{a/c}{b/d}$$

This OR will estimate the prevalence proportion of diabetes among those with the mutation divided by the prevalence proportion among those without the mutation, but the problem is that we use prevalence data and prevalence is a function of incidence and disease duration. We are studying onset of diabetes or MS and surviving with diabetes or MS at the same time, and we cannot disentangle whether the genetic variant increases the risk of getting the disease or whether it improves survival. At least we need additional data to obtain that information, and our estimates need not reflect relative risks if the exposure is associated with disease duration. If the exposure (a genetic variant) has prognostic implications a relative prevalence measure is a function of both etiologic and prognostic factors. We may get unbiased estimates of relative risks even when using prevalent cases if the exposures under study have no prognostic importance. If the genetic variant increases life expectancy for MS cases, the OR would be high, even when being unrelated to incidence, and the naïve (and wrong) conclusion could be that the genetic variant causes MS.

It may be difficult to recruit incidence cases if the disease has a high mortality, especially if you need to interview the cases. Assume that you want to study whether physical fitness prevents myocardial infarctions (MI) and you have to interview the cases about their physical activity in the past. You cannot interview cases in the acute phase of their MI – you have to wait until their health improves, and in this time period the most seriously ill patients will die. Assume, for the sake of the argument, that physical exercise has no impact on the incidence of MI (it has) but improves the prognosis (decreases short-term mortality), then the underlying cohort could produce data as in Table 10.7.

Table 10.7 A cohort study on physical exercise and myocardial infarctions (MI)

Physical exercise	N	MI	Death	Cases for interview
Yes	10,000	50	10	40
No	10,000	50	20	30

$$RR = \frac{50/10,000}{50/10,000} = 1.0$$

And a case–cohort study taken from this cohort among survivors would look like Table 10.8.

Table 10.8 A case–control study based on data on survivors from Table 10.7

Physical exercise	Cases	Controls
Yes	40	35
No	30	35
All	70	70

$$OR = \frac{40/30}{35/35} = 1.33$$

The OR apparently wrongly indicates, according to the conditions we have set, that physical exercise increases the risk of MI. The reason is that we did not recruit all incidence cases but only the survivors. Had we recruited all incidence cases the table would look like Table 10.9.

Table 10.9 A case–control study based on data from baseline, Table 10.7

Physical exercise	Cases	Controls
Yes	50	50
No	50	50
All	100	100

$$OR = \frac{50/50}{50/50} = 1.00$$

In principle we could have obtained unbiased results if we had included proxy responders to replace the deceased MI patients, for example close relatives, but by doing so we rely on low-quality exposure data and may get information-biased results.

In brief, measures of association are based upon comparisons of disease risk for the exposed and disease risk for the unexposed. We use the underlying population experience during a given follow-up period to obtain this information whether we perform a follow-up study or a case–control study. In setting up a case–control study there are different ways of sampling this population experience depending upon which measure of association we take an interest in: a relative risk, incidence rate ratios, or relative prevalence proportions.

When to Do a Case–Control Study?

Since case–control sampling aims at maximizing the amount of information from the underlying population at the lowest possible cost, the case–control study is usually the design of choice if the disease under study is rare, if conditions for doing the study are fulfilled, and if the exposure under study is not too rare. The most important of these conditions is the ability to get valid exposure data on the putative causes of the disease. Genetic factors that are stable over time would fulfill this criterion but if you take an interest in gene expression over time it may be different. It is more difficult to get valid data for exposures that change over time and especially for exposures that have to be recalled by the participants, such as dietary data. Eating habits change over time and cannot be recalled with any kind of precision more than days or perhaps weeks back in time. It will also be difficult to recall medicine intake back in time, unless the medicine has been used regularly over long time periods, such as insulin. If valid records exist and are available for study, like medical records or records of occupational exposures, these may not only replace uncertain recalls but also provide more comparable data for cases and controls. In a case–control study on use of mobile phones and brain cancer it will probably be too uncertain to rely on recall of phone use back in time. The magnitude of mobile phone use is difficult to recall and it may be impossible to obtain the same degree of accuracy in recall (symmetry in recall) among cases and controls. The cases have a disease that may interfere with cognitive functions and they may have incentives to exaggerate phone use that are not present among controls. If billing records are available from phone companies, the study may provide comparable exposure data over time and these data may be preferable although they are incomplete or even wrong in some situations. Billing records may lack data on incoming calls and will not indicate how the phone was used or who used it.

A case–control study is usually much more vulnerable to selection bias related to non-responders than a follow-up study because both the exposure and the disease may play a role when participants decide to accept or decline the invitation to take part in the study. Low response rates can easily make results from a case–control study unreliable and misleading.

A population-based case–control study is a study using a source population defined a priori by certain geographical boundaries, but if only a few of the cases accept the invitation to participate the "population-based aspect" becomes misleading and it may be better to let the source population be defined by the case series (to use a case-defined (secondary) source population).

Since sampling in a case–control study focuses upon diseased and a sample from their source population, the population they came from, the case–control study usually focuses on a single disease but provides an open opportunity to study a set of different exposures as putative determinants. Case–control studies are for that reason often based on interviews using lengthy questionnaires. Genetic association studies usually screen for a large number of gene variants. A case–control study is a study "looking for a cause of the disease" whereas the follow-up study addresses an exposure "looking for a disease to occur."

A case–control study has the potential of producing information much faster than a follow-up study, especially if there is a long induction and latency time between the exposures and the onset of the disease. When cases and controls are recruited, the induction and latency time is already over since you sample cases with the disease. In a cohort study with prospective data we would have to wait for this time period to pass and therefore the exposure has to have been present in the population long enough for the exposures to cause the disease under study. If we want to study whether a newly established technology causes cancer after 5–10 years of incubation and latency time, we may, however, do better by setting up a cohort to harvest the information as soon as it is available, since a case–control study cannot provide data before the cases start to emerge from the exposure we take an interest in.

References

1. Nagel E (ed.). John Stuart Mill's Philosophy of Scientific Method. Hafner Press, New York, 1950.
2. Miettinen OS. Subject selection in case-referent studies with a secondary base. J Chronic Dis 1987;40(2):186–187.

Chapter 11
The Cross-Sectional Study

In a cross-sectional study, all in a given population or a random sample from this population define the source population. The disease and its possible determinants are all recorded at a given point in time. This introduces a temporal ambiguity in the possible cause–effect association and for this reason most *cross-sectional studies* have survey purposes that are only descriptive. We use cross-sectional studies to estimate, e.g., the prevalence of depression or the prevalence of having shift work. We may, however, also use the design to study stable determinants, like genetic factors, if these factors only impact etiology and not the prognosis. Assume a cross-sectional study gives the results stated in Table 11.1.

$$RP = \frac{300/2{,}300}{700/8{,}700} = 1.62$$

Table 11.1 A cross-sectional study on hormones and breast cancer

Use of hormone replacement therapy (HRT)	Breast cancer		
	Yes	No	All
Yes	300	2,000	2,300
No	700	8,000	8,700
All	1,000	10,000	11,000

This prevalence ratio may reflect that HRT causes breast cancer or that HRT prolongs survival (improves the prognosing of breast cancer) or that breast cancer leads to an increased use of HRT (unlikely). And of course the association could be caused by bias, confounding, or chance.

Cross-sectional studies (or surveys) are important in monitoring disease frequencies or risk factors over time, but they play a limited role in analytical epidemiology addressing non-genetic determinant diseases.

When estimating disease occurrence in a cross-sectional study it should be recognized that the duration of the disease affects the probability of being sampled. A person with pneumonia lasting 10 weeks has 10 times the probability of being in the cross-sectional sample than a person with pneumonia lasting 1 week. Prevalence data are *length biased* when we compare them with incidence data.

J. Olsen et al., *An Introduction to Epidemiology for Health Professionals*, Springer Series on Epidemiology and Health 1, DOI 10.1007/978-1-4419-1497-2_11, © Springer Science+Business Media, LLC 2010

Chapter 12
The Randomized Controlled Trial (RCT)

Sometimes it may be possible to set up an experimental study, especially in clinical epidemiology. A new treatment may be compared with the standard treatment using one or more features of a randomized trial. The key, and obligatory, feature in the randomized trial is *randomization*, which is the allocation of two (or more) treatments that are to be compared by letting this allocation depend on the result of a random process like flipping a coin. By doing so, we let the selection of treatment be independent of the disease characteristics and other potential confounding factors. We obtain (in the long run) that the two groups will have the same treatment results if the two treatments are equally good or equally bad and all comply with the protocolled treatment allocation. Randomization is of crucial importance in avoiding what is called "confounding by indication" – the indication for treatment may confound the estimate of the treatment effect – since there are hopefully good reasons for using one particular treatment rather than another. Randomization will, in the long run, remove confounding, including confounding by indication and confounding by unknown factors. A perfectly designed and conducted randomized trial will, if repeated over and over again, approach the true causal association between the exposure and the disease under study. It is unfortunately much easier to design a "perfect" RCT than to conduct one.

The second element is *blinding*, i.e., using unlabeled treatments that cannot be distinguished from each other. They are packed in similar containers, look alike, taste alike if they are going to be eaten, etc. Blinding is used to avoid differential misclassifications of, for example, side effects or treatment effects. Double blinding means that neither the patient nor the researcher knows which treatment has been given. Triple blinding indicates that also the person analyzing the data is blinded until all main results are estimated with coded values for treatment.

The outcome (estimated treatment effect) of a trial is a function of the natural history of the disease, the possible biased reporting by the patients, doctors, and statisticians, and the possible treatment effect. Use of randomization, blinding, and *placebo* (an inactive treatment) or comparison with the best available treatment makes it possible to isolate the treatment effect. If we run a large randomized trial where the expected natural history of the disease does not differ between the compared groups and if blinding makes measurement errors similar in both groups, then

J. Olsen et al., *An Introduction to Epidemiology for Health Professionals*,
Springer Series on Epidemiology and Health 1, DOI 10.1007/978-1-4419-1497-2_12,
© Springer Science+Business Media, LLC 2010

we may be in a situation where we are entitled to say that a significant difference in prognosis probably reflects a treatment effect, but not more than that. Unfortunately, complete compliance to the protocol is seldom seen. People stop taking medicine they do not believe works or they start taking something else.

Randomized controlled trials are usually based on informed consent, and the sequence of a trial could be as in Fig. 12.1.

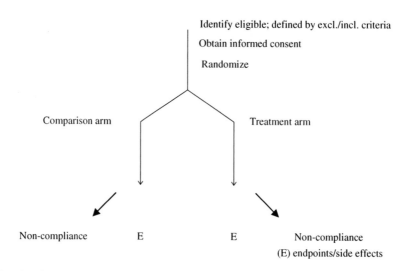

Fig. 12.1   Structure of an RCT

The randomized trial is a follow-up study where the exposed and unexposed cohorts are selected from the same pool of eligible candidates. They have the disease to be treated and they are of the desired age and have other characteristics of importance for the treatment. If they say yes to taking part in the trial (many do not), they are then randomized to one of the two (or possibly more) arms. It is important to make sure that the information fully explains the time they need to devote to the study, the procedures they have to go through and possible risks associated with the treatment. During follow-up the investigator has to record compliance to the research protocol and often an independent monitoring committee has to follow possible side effects and other deviations from the expected outcomes.

Data are then usually analyzed according to the principle we call *intention to treat* or "as randomized so analyzed." All comparisons are made between the randomized groups, regardless of whether they followed the treatment or not. The reason for not comparing those who actually followed the protocol (this analysis is called *according to protocol*), is that participants made the decision to comply or not to comply and we may lose comparability obtained at randomization by the selection bias this may entail.

Analyzing data according to the "intention to treat" principle is no guarantee against bias when we try to estimate the treatment effects. It may, in fact, be a guarantee for bias. If a large number of people do not follow the protocol then we underestimate the treatment effects (and side effects), and if many do not comply the comparison may be of little clinical relevance. Furthermore, intention to treat analysis requires that we have the key endpoint data for those who left the study, which may not always be the case.

Since a randomized trial is an intervention where we impose an exposure we must accept the responsibilities that it entails. Randomized trials are usually not an option if we want to study harmful exposures, like an environmental exposure or risky lifestyle factors. In order to do a trial to compare different treatments we need to be of the belief that these treatments may turn out to be equally good or bad. If we believe one treatment is better than the other the trial is unethical; the principle of *equipoise* is then violated.

Randomized trials usually have to be relatively large to be worth doing since small trials do not guarantee comparability between treatment groups. Flipping a coin 10 times only occasionally produces 50% heads and 50% tails. Flipping a coin 1,000 times will yield results much closer to this expectation.

Analyzing data from a randomized trial is similar to analyzing data from any other follow-up study measuring relative or absolute measures of association. Besides these measures, you will find a measure such as "numbers needed to treat (1 divided by the difference in risk between the two groups)." A trial on folate use to prevent neural tube defects in high-risk pregnant women showed the results given in Table 12.1 [1].

Table 12.1   Preventing neural tube defects (NTD) by using folic acid

Exposure/folic acid	Number of children	Number with neural tube defects at birth
+	593	6
−	602	21

$$\text{Relative prevalence ratio} = \frac{6/593}{21/602} = 0.29$$

$$\text{Relative prevalence difference (RPD)} = 21/602 - 6/593 = 0.025$$

$$\text{Numbers needed to treat } 1/\text{RPD} = 1/0.025 = 40$$

The estimates show that folate prevents a number of neural tube defects. The prevalence proportion is about 70% lower among those who received folate than among those who did not (the prevalence proportion drops from 0.0035 to 0.0010). About 40 of these high-risk women (women who had a previous child with a neural tube defect) have to receive folate supplementation to prevent one case with a neural tube defect to be born – a remarkable cost-effective preventive treatment since folate is cheap and has few, if any, side effects in the doses needed to obtain a preventive effect [1].

Reference

1. MRC Vitamin Study Research Group. Prevention of neural tube defects: results of the Medical Research Council Vitamin Study. Lancet 1991;338(8760):131–137.

Chapter 13
Analytical Epidemiology in Public Health

Since the public health epidemiologist focuses on determinants of disease or ways of preventing diseases, an experimental study is often not an option for ethical reasons, although it may be possible to remove an exposure in a randomized trial on, e.g., smoking cessation. The public health epidemiologist will need to know more about non-experimental design options and how to use available data for research. The public health epidemiologist will often use *secondary data* (data generated for a different purpose, like death certificates, existing monitoring data of air pollution, employment roosters), and he or she will have to be familiar with how the data were generated and the limitations that may imply.

The public health epidemiologist should provide information on changes in morbidity and mortality and be able to address changes related to unemployment, changes in health care or rapid changes in important risk factors such as obesity, emerging epidemics, and more. It is important to have broad and general data on health in a population to set priorities right.

The public health epidemiologist is also expected to be able to go beyond simple vital statistics and to identify patterns in morbidity or mortality that can be used to generate new hypotheses about possible causes of diseases. A public health epidemiologist will know that a hypothesis also has to be evaluated within an epidemiologic context. Does the disease follow a pattern that at least does not contradict the hypothesis? If you claim that mobile phone use increases a specific form of brain cancer you would at least expect this cancer to increase over time since the exposure is increasing rapidly over time. You will expect to see this increase to be strongest in age groups and populations that use the phone most often once they have accumulated sufficient exposure time to onset the disease. The public health epidemiologist should also be familiar with more design options than has been described in the previous text.

Population-based case–control sampling, for example, is difficult and vulnerable to a variety of different sources of error and the public health epidemiologist should know about important design alternatives like the case-crossover study [1] that in some situations is less bias prone. The idea is simple, namely that for an exposure that changes over time, like diet, physical exercise, and intake of medicine, individual disease experience can be used to examine associations with diseases that have a short induction and latency time. The person may observe that migraine is more

J. Olsen et al., *An Introduction to Epidemiology for Health Professionals*,
Springer Series on Epidemiology and Health 1, DOI 10.1007/978-1-4419-1497-2_13,
© Springer Science+Business Media, LLC 2010

frequent following intake of red wine than in time periods without this exposure (the incidence rate is higher in exposed time than in unexposed time). In the case-crossover design we try to combine this experience from several people to make a common estimate from a group of cases. A larger sample is needed if the disease is rare.

The Case-Crossover Study

The *case-crossover study* starts with identifying cases and only cases are used (it is a case-only study). We record whether the exposure was present shortly before the onset of the disease and in a pre-specified reference time period. To make this less abstract let us use data from a published study to illustrate the design.

Redelmeier and Tibshirani [2] took an interest in studying the association between using mobile phones and car accidents. They identified drivers who had a car accident and recorded use of mobile phones in a 10-min time period leading up to the accident and for a reference 10-min time period on a similar day of the week before. They recorded mobile phone use if the individuals were driving and using the mobile phone at that time. Given these data, they classified all cases according to Table 13.1.

Table 13.1 The four possible exposure profiles of cases

	Use of mobile phone	
Type	Reference 10 min	Before accident 10 min
1	Yes	Yes
2	Yes	No
3	No	Yes
4	No	No

All information on risk comes from type 2 and type 3 people. A type 2 response indicates a protective effect and a type 3 response a harmful effect of using the phone while driving. It turns out that the estimate of RR in this simple example is obtained by calculating the total number of type 3 cases and dividing it with the total number of type 2 cases. We use only drivers that are discordant for the exposure in the two time periods:

$$RR = \frac{\sum type3}{\sum type2}$$

Table 13.2 shows results from the study, and the results indicate that use of mobile phones increases the risk of accidents about fourfold.

The table shows, perhaps as expected, that young people with short driving experience have the highest relative risks of having an accident when using a mobile phone. It was more unexpected that using hands-free sets carried as high a risk as

Table 13.2 Relative risk of a motor vehicle collision following use of mobile phones, according to selected characteristics [2]

Characteristics	Relative risk (95%) confidence limits
All subjects	4.3 (3.0–6.5)
Age (year)	
<25	6.5 (2.2–∞)
25–39	4.4 (2.8–8.8)
40–54	3.6 (2.1–8.7)
>55	3.3 (1.5–∞)
Sex	
Male	4.1 (2.8–6.4)
Female	4.8 (2.6–14.0)
Driving experience (year)	
0–9	6.2 (2.8–25.0)
10–19	4.3 (2.6–10.0)
20–29	3.0 (1.7–7.0)
≥30	4.4 (2.1–17.0)
Type of mobile phone	
Hand-held	3.9 (2.7–6.1)
Hands-free	5.9 (2.9–24.0)

hand-held phones. The results may even indicate that the use of hands-free sets carries a higher risk, but the confidence intervals (CI) show that these estimates come with statistical uncertainties.

By making cases their own controls we adjust for all confounders that remain stable over the time period of study in this case up to a week (like driving skills or genetic factors and in most cases car safety); we even obtain much better control over these factors than in any other designs, including the randomized controlled design, and we obtain better control of genetic factors than we could obtain in a twin study. We are closer to the counterfactual ideal than in most other designs for these time-stable factors. But there are also limitations. Were the driving conditions similar at the two occasions? Perhaps the use of a mobile phone was done to inform about delays and heavy traffic? These traffic conditions could be component causes of the accidents rather than phone use and of course we have to make sure that the phone calls were done before the accident and not to call for help after the accident (reverse causation).

References

1. Maclure M. The case-crossover design: a method for studying transient effects on the risk of acute events. Am J Epidemiol 1991;133:144–153.
2. Redelmeier D, Tibshirani RJ. Association between cellular-telephone calls and motor vehicle collisions. N Engl J Med 1997;336(7):453–458.

Chapter 14
Analytical Epidemiology in Genetic Epidemiology

Disentangling the Basis for Clustering in Families

The recurrence of diseases or correlation in traits can, through studies of adoptees, twins, and half-sibs, provide information about the causes of familial clustering. Other kinds of family studies cannot separate the effect of shared environment and shared genes.

Adoption Studies

For logistic reasons, adoption studies are fewer and usually smaller than other family studies. Nevertheless, *adoption studies* have had a substantial impact on the *nature–nurture debate* for a number of traits because these studies have produced remarkable results. Adoption studies use the fact that adoptees share genetic variants with their biological parents but not the parents' environment, and they share the environment to some extent, but not gene variants, with their adoptive families. Among the most notable findings from adoption studies is Heston's 1966 study [1], where he showed that among 47 children who had schizophrenic mothers and who were put up for adoption 5 developed schizophrenia, while none of the 50 control adoptees developed schizophrenia. Although the sample size is small, the study very convincingly indicated that schizophrenia has a strong genetic component. A strong intrauterine component could also be an explanation but twin studies reveal much higher concordance rates in monozygotic twins compared to dizygotic twins (see below), again suggesting genetic factors as the major factor in susceptibility to schizophrenia [2]. Another intriguing finding that surprised many was a Danish adoption study of BMI [3]. This study showed that the BMI of adoptees correlated more with the BMI of their biological relatives than that of their adoptive relatives, indicating a strong genetic or early life component to variation in body composition in settings with no shortage of food supply.

J. Olsen et al., *An Introduction to Epidemiology for Health Professionals*,
Springer Series on Epidemiology and Health 1, DOI 10.1007/978-1-4419-1497-2_14,
© Springer Science+Business Media, LLC 2010

Twin Studies

In humans two types of twinning occur: *monozygotic (identical) twins*, who share all their genetic material, and *dizygotic (fraternal) twins*, who on average share 50% of their genes by descent like non-twin siblings. A *twin study* of a condition/disease in its simplest form is based on a comparison of monozygotic and dizygotic concordance rates (i.e., the probability that a twin has the condition under study given that the co-twin has it), corresponding to the recurrence risk described on page 38–39. A significantly higher concordance rate in monozygotic than in dizygotic twins indicates that genetic factors play a role in the etiology of the disease. For continuous traits, correlations are used instead of concordance rates. The twin study does not identify specific genes that affect the trait but rather assesses the overall effect of genetic factors: the degree to which differences in the phenotype are attributable to genetic differences between people. To estimate the *heritability* of a trait (i.e., the proportion of the population variance attributable to genetic variation) twin data can be analyzed using standard biometric models. A number of recent developments in twin methodology have taken place based on the incorporation of genotypes. This enables twin models to estimate how much of the genetic variation is due to variation in a specific gene. The classic twin methodology is based on genetic theory and the fundamental idea is that a higher degree of similarity for a trait within monozygotic twins compared to dizygotic twins is attributable to the higher degree of genetic similarity in monozygotic twins.

Twin studies of Alzheimer's disease (not early onset) show that a co-twin of an affected monozygotic twin has a 60–80% risk of becoming affected, while the risk is 30–40% if the pair is dizygotic. For Parkinson's disease the corresponding numbers are about 5% for both monozygotic and dizygotic twins. This is compatible with a strong genetic influence on Alzheimer's disease while most etiological factors for Parkinson's disease are likely to be identified in the environment some genetic risks for Parkinson's disease are now known.

Twin studies are not theoretical models such as the component causal model. Under such models it is easy to argue that all diseases are 100% genetically and 100% environmentally determined because it is hard to imagine any disease that does not have both environmental and genetic components. However, in the practical research process of identifying factors influencing disease occurrence in a given setting at a given time the classic twin study is very useful. Twin studies can point toward identifiable causes of variation in a given population, e.g., to which degree it is likely that genetic differences between people play a major role for the occurrence of that disease in that population, as seen in the Alzheimer's disease occurrence described above.

Half-Sib Studies

In countries with population registers it is possible, on a nationwide level, to identify individuals who have changed their spouse or residence (or other environmental factors). Information from these registers can be used to set up a study that is particularly well suited for studying nature–nurture effects on reproductive outcomes or diseases in early childhood [4].

Interpretation of Heritability

Twin and adoption studies suggest that a wide variety of phenotypes have a genetic component to their etiology. Note that heritability estimates are time and population specific, i.e., the overall influence of genetic factors depends on the amount of environmental variance in the study population and vice versa. If, for example, more equal access to favorable living conditions and health care is introduced in a population, this is likely to decrease the environmental variance and hence increase the proportion of the total variation attributable to genetic factors (the heritability). On the other hand, an increase in the environmental variance as seen in modern societies can also provide the opportunity for genetic effects to become expressed.

A substantial heritability for a trait suggests that it may be possible to identify specific genetic variants that influence the trait. The chance of identifying gene variants affecting a trait through genetic association or family studies depends on the number of gene variants and the size of their effect.

Estimating effects in genetic epidemiology:

- What are the specific genetic variants and environmental factors influencing the trait or disease?
- How do the environmental and genetic factors interact?

Exposure–Disease Associations Through Studies of Relatives

Nearly all lung cancers occur in smokers. Although overwhelming evidence exists for the health-damaging effects of smoking from observational studies and animal studies it could be claimed that what we observe is just an association between smoking and lung cancer and that we do not know whether it is causal or a result of confounding, e.g., genetic confounding. While this today may seem farfetched, one of the leading bio-statisticians, Sir Ronald Fisher (1890–1962), actually argued that smoking in itself did not cause lung cancer but that certain genetic variants increase the liability to smoke as well as the liability to develop lung cancer, and he was not alone in holding this belief at that time. Doll and Hill recognized this possibility in their landmark paper on smoking and lung cancer from 1950 [5].

Twin studies may shed light on this hypothesis and similar (unlikely) hypotheses that familial-shared environmental factors would be the basis for the association. The informative twin pairs are discordant pairs, like in the case-crossover study (i.e., twin pairs where one twin is a smoker and the other is not). If the smoking–lung cancer association is caused by genetic factors, we would not expect the smoking co-twin to get lung cancer more often among monozygotic twins than the non-smoking co-twin because the two twins share all genetic factors. For dizygotic twins we would expect a weaker association than observed in the general population because we partly control for genetic factors (dizygotic twins share, like siblings, about 50% of their genes). If the smoking–lung cancer association is not due to genetic or other familial factors we will expect to see that the smoking co-twins have the highest lung cancer risk regardless of zygosity. Studies of siblings correspond genetically to studies of dizygotic twins. Sibling studies benefit from the fact that sibships are much more common than twins. Furthermore, many twins have infertile parents as twinning may be a result of infertility treatment they received, although this is only a potential problem for younger cohorts of twins.

While the above example is mostly of historic interest, this design can also be used to address some of the important contemporary topics in epidemiology: There is evidence that an association exists between fetal growth and later life health outcomes, such as blood pressure and cardiovascular mortality. The key question is, however, whether fetal nourishment or other factors such as genes or socioeconomic conditions cause the association. Some studies suggest that socioeconomic confounding cannot explain the association between fetal growth and cardiovascular mortality, but there is evidence that genetic polymorphism can affect both fetal growth and later insulin regulation. Analysis of twin pairs provides no strong evidence that the smallest twin at birth later has the highest blood pressure, suggesting that at least part of the association can be explained by familial factors including genetic factors and the rearing environment [6].

Gene–Environment Interaction

It is difficult to imagine diseases that are not at least in part due to interactions between genetic and environmental factors. A clear example of *gene–environment interaction* is G6PD deficiency. This is an X-linked trait of the enzyme *glucose-6-phosphate dehydrogenase* deficiency that facilitates energy metabolism in cells (like red blood cells) and helps protect the cell from oxidative damage. Defects in the enzyme that are genetically determined are extremely common (~5% worldwide) and can result in hemolysis and anemia if the affected are exposed to certain nutritional insults such as Fava beans or pharmacologic agents including some antibiotics and antimalarials. Thus individuals with a risk genotype are normal in the absence of an environmental exposure. This is an example where the causal field model fits the observation. The strength between the genetic factor and the disease depends upon the prevalence of the dietary factors and medicine use. By avoiding these environmental exposures we make sure the causal field is not completed.

Also the common ApoE-4 polymorphism, which has been shown to be a risk factor for cardiovascular diseases and Alzheimer's disease, seems to be involved in gene–environment interaction making the ApoE-4 carrier more susceptible to environmental exposures. For example, an increased risk of chronic brain injury after head trauma has been observed for individuals who carry the ApoE-4 gene variant, compared to non-ApoE-4 carriers.

A huge challenge to gene–environment interaction studies is the *multiple comparison* problem. With approximately 20,000 genes already identified, many having several variants, an enormous number of possible gene–environment interactions can be studied. One reasonable strategy is testing of biologically plausible interactions and replication of positive findings in large studies.

Cross-Sectional Studies of Genetic Polymorphisms

If we did not already know from vital statistics that males have substantially higher mortality than females throughout life, we could get information about this from a cross-sectional population-based study. We would see that in many countries the distribution of males to females would be approximately 1:1 at birth while it is about 1:2 at age 85 and 1:4 or even 1:5 at age 100 in many settings. Similarly some genetic variants, e.g., ApoE-4, are "weeded out" with age, indicating that they are associated with increased mortality. Interference from such cross-sectional studies is dependent on a stable population with little migration into the population. Remote islands will therefore often be very well suited for such cross-sectional age-dependency studies while immigrant countries like the USA and Australia are less suited.

Incorporation of Genetic Variables in Epidemiologic Studies

Advances in technology frequently enable new and more powerful analytic approaches to disease causality. While it has been possible to include variability in genes into studies of epidemiology since the discovery of the human blood group antigens in the early 1900s, there has been a remarkable advance in using genetic variables in the last few years as DNA sequencing and related technologies make it feasible to study up to 1 million variants per individual on thousands of cases and controls at practical costs. Two general options are currently available for large epidemiologic studies. One is directly hypothesis driven and involves choosing a modest number of variants for study when the underlying biology/physiology of the risk alleles is already known or highly suspected. This is called the *candidate gene approach* and might be used in a setting of building on a known effect such as the role of ApoE variants in dementia or cardiovascular disease or genes such as the *N*-acetyltransferases that are critical in cigarette smoke detoxification. Selecting for study variants in genes of known biological function enables the investigator to add a powerful new variable to the analysis and limits the problems that arise from multiple comparisons and the attendant issue of false positive results (type 1 errors). If we has no strong candidates or wishes to investigate the role of common variants without a prior hypothesis as to what genes those variants might be present in one can use the *genome wide association study* (*GWAS*). In 2007 advances in both technology for variant detection (a range of "DNA chips") and analytic advances in how to address the type 1 error problem resulted in an explosion of GWAS studies leading to the identification possible of gene variants contributing to a wide range of common, complex disorders. The technology allows the study of up to 1 million single nucleotide polymorphisms (SNPs) as well as 1 million *copy number variants (CNVs)* on a single individual for less than 500 Euros. This technology takes advantage of the observation that common human genetic variation is located in blocks where tens or even hundreds of variants in physical proximity on a chromosome each have their individual alleles inherited in a manner highly correlated with the alleles of nearby SNPs [7]. Thus any one *SNP* can serve as a surrogate marker for many others, making it practical to provide coverage of an entire genome with a few hundred thousand SNPs and CNVs. As the cost of the assays is expected to drop further such approaches are now a standard tool in genetic epidemiologic studies. There are a few caveats. First, the approach is only effective when common variants contributing to disease can be detected by virtue of their disease association. While this is true for some single-gene disorders (cystic fibrosis, for example) as well as complex traits (breast cancer and many others) it is not true for all disorders (PKU and hypertension seem to be exceptions). In these disorders a genetic component may still be very active but a large number of different alleles may be contributing so that no common variant can be detected by association. These multiple allele disorders can be solved by DNA sequencing, and while the cost of DNA sequencing is low it remains costly enough that it is not yet in routine use for epidemiologic studies that lack a hypothesis for a specific region to examine. Next, because of the enormity of the multiple comparisons (a P value of $<10E\text{-}7$ is required to meet Bonferroni expectations) there are many signals that may require evaluation so that replication in independent populations for positive results is now an expectation for any such study to be accepted. Nonetheless, GWAS studies are now a component of most large epidemiologic efforts, and plans for obtaining material for DNA should be a standard plan for any study in which a genetic variable might be active.

References

1. Heston LL. Psychiatric disorders in foster home reared children of schizophrenic mothers. Br J Psychiatry 1966;112(489):819–825.
2. Plomin R, Owen MJ, McGuffin P. The genetic basis of complex human behaviors. Science 1994 Jun 17;264(5166):1733–1739. Review.
3. Sørensen TI, Holst C, Stunkard AJ. Adoption study of environmental modifications of the genetic influences on obesity. Int Obes Relat Metab Disord 1998;22(1):73–81.
4. Olsen J, Schmidt MM, Christensen K. Evaluation of nature-nurture impact on reproductive health using half-siblings. Epidemiology 1997;8(1):6–11.
5. Doll R, Hill AB. Smoking and carcinoma of the lung. Br Med J 1950;4682:739–748.
6. Kujala UM, Kaprio J, Koskenvuo M. Modifiable risk factors as predictors of all-cause mortality: the roles of genetics and childhood environment. Am J Epidemiol 2002;156(11):985–993.
7. Christensen K, Murray JC. What genome-wide association studies can do for medicine. N Engl J Med 2007 Mar 15;356(11):1094–1097.

Chapter 15
Analytical Epidemiology in Clinical Epidemiology

Common Designs Used to Estimate Associations

In order to evaluate interventions or diagnostic procedures a *randomized clinical trial* (RCT) is the most accepted way. However, there are certain limitations:

1. It may be problematic to generalize the results from an RCT into normal clinical practice.
   RCTs are normally restricted to selected patient groups, often excluding children, pregnant women, and geriatric patients.
2. Long-term effects. RCTs are normally costly undertakings, which means that a follow-up exceeding 1–2 years is very uncommon and side effects may well take longer to develop.
3. Studying rare events requires very large studies. Clinical studies encompassing more than 500 in each arm are rare, which means that events with a frequency of 1 out of 200 or less will seldom be detected in the statistical analyses.
4. Interactions with other diseases and/or other drugs, etc. Thus, in many instances one has to use other designs in order to estimate effects or side effects.

Case-Reports and Cross-Sectional Studies

Most medical students or junior doctors will sometimes encounter a senior colleague who will tell her/him with conviction that once upon a time he/she had a patient who had both diseases A and B and reacted badly to drug C and consequently treatment D will be the only appropriate choice for this patient. The senior colleague is then inferring from a case-report, and caution is recommended. Further, results from different cross-sectional studies have often been interpreted without taking the time sequence of events into consideration.

One example comes from the Third International Conference on *Pernicious Anaemia* in Stockholm in August 1937. Pernicious anemia had up to then been regarded as a malignancy with a hematological picture impossible to distinguish from leukemia. Now it could be cured by giving patients B12. Dr. Birger Strandell,

J. Olsen et al., *An Introduction to Epidemiology for Health Professionals*,
Springer Series on Epidemiology and Health 1, DOI 10.1007/978-1-4419-1497-2_15,
© Springer Science+Business Media, LLC 2010

a Swedish internist, who had used data from the newly established regional cancer registry in order to assess the long-term effects following cure for pernicious anemia, demonstrated that the patients had a very high risk for gastric cancer. He inferred that patients with pernicious anemia were at an increased risk of gastric cancer which had clinical implications. He even had this report accepted in the *Journal of Nordic Medicine* (in Swedish with an abstract in German). However, the next speaker was Professor Karsner from Cleveland, Ohio, who presented the results from a study performed at his clinic [1]. It was a cross-sectional study including more than 1,000 individuals with pernicious anemia had been diagnosed, none of whom had gastric cancer at the time of diagnosis of pernicious anemia, and he wrote in *JAMA* that there was no association between pernicious anemia and gastric cancer. Although this was published before impact factors existed *JAMA* evidently was more widely read than the *Journal of Nordic Medicine*, and the results from Cleveland became the accepted truth until the end of the 1970s. We know now that pernicious anemia can lead to gastric cancer, and cross-sectional studies that do not take into account the temporal dimension can produce misleading results and misguide clinical practice.

Case–Control Studies

Screening is suitable for evaluation in observational studies, and randomized clinical trials will in most instances be very difficult to conduct. An RCT may provide information produced under ideal circumstances (efficacy) that need not represent what happens when screening becomes a routine procedure (effectiveness). The outcome of interest is often relatively rare even in high-risk populations, and long-term effects, often after decades, are of special interest. A good example on how to evaluate a possible impact of screening for *colorectal cancer* is a study from the Kaiser Permanente Medical Care program published in 1992 [2].

Two hundred and sixty-one members who died of cancer of the rectum or distal colon between 1971 and 1988 were used as cases and 868 controls were matched on sex and age. Sigmoidoscopy performed up to 10 years before the diagnosis of a cancer was the screening test and the authors demonstrated a 60% reduction in mortality from rectal or distal colon cancer following screening. This reduction in mortality could be due to other exposures such as lifestyle factors or medication. In order to study if confounding explained the results 268 subjects who had died from colon cancer above the reach of sigmoidoscopy and 268 controls showed no difference in the use of sigmoidoscopy between cases and controls. Finding a similar colon cancer mortality in these two groups indicates that intervention with sigmoidoscopy was related to this reduction in cause-specific mortality in humans within the reach of sigmoidoscopy. Similar results have been found in randomized trials.

Cohort Studies

A letter to the editor in 1932 [3] made the case that the adherences following a *perforated appendix* in females would affect their long-term fertility. The author therefore recommended a liberal attitude for abdominal exploration at the suspicion of appendicitis in young females. This notion was enforced by different case series and became the accepted truth leading to a female predominance of appendectomies, especially in the younger age groups. This practice was challenged for the first time in the 1990s in a study from Sweden [4]. Close to 10,000 women subjected to appendectomy under the age of 15 between 1964 and 1983 were compared to 47,000 women who had no appendectomy before the age of 15. The authors demonstrated that with the exception of women who had been appendectomized with a normal appendix there was no difference in the fertility between those with a perforated appendix and those with an appendicitis that did not perforate (Fig. 15.1).

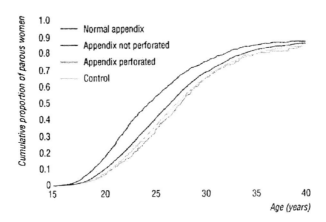

Fig. 15.1 Age-specific rates of first birth among women who underwent appendicectomy before age 15 and among age-matched controls according to life table analysis. Figure shows average birth rate in a given 2-year age interval

The somewhat lower age at first birth among those with a normal appendix is not surprising as these women probably to some extent were more sexually active at an earlier age than the rest, leading to infections mimicking appendicitis. The publication of this study combined with better diagnostic instruments for appendicitis has since then resulted in a more even sex distribution among the appendectomized, for instance in 2006 there were 5,358 appendectomies in males compared to 5,039 in females in Sweden [5].

Randomized Clinical Trials (RCTs)

A randomized clinical trial is a cohort study. There is, however, one major component in the random clinical trial which gives it a certain advantage to the observational study, namely *randomization.*

A correctly conducted large randomized trial will reduce confounding. If the study is large enough the distribution of potential confounders will be similar in both arms.

However, two quality indicators of the study should always be assessed by the reader:

1. Analyzing data according to "intention to treat" is the key. Otherwise selection bias will be of concern.
2. Blinding of the treatment among those assessing the outcome. Otherwise the results can be subject to differential misclassification.

In the 1980s laparoscopic cholecystectomy surgery (surgery through a scope to remove gallbladder stones) was introduced. This new method was deemed to be superior with regard to the postoperative period compared to open surgery. It was therefore considered unethical as well as unnecessary to perform clinical trials. Observational studies were difficult to conduct following this procedure due to confounding by indication, i.e., confounding by the reason for using a specific type of surgery. The first randomized clinical trial was therefore conducted as late as in 1992. Two hundred patients were included and randomization took place in the operation room after which the procedure was performed either laparoscopically or as an open operation. Identical wound dressings were applied in both groups, and both caretakers and patients were blinded to the type of operation. Drains were usually removed on the first postoperative day, patient control analgesics were discontinued at the discretion of a patient, and oral analgesia was given if necessary. The patients were interviewed in the out-patient clinic by a research nurse who was unaware of the operation procedure, and the wounds were checked by a surgeon in a separate room. The authors demonstrated that a laparoscopic cholecystectomy takes longer compared to open surgery and does not have an advantage in terms of hospital stay or postoperative recovery. These findings were unexpected but have so far had no impact on the patterns of operations.

In conclusion, observational studies in combination with randomized, clinical trials are the main method to evaluate new techniques, interventions, and diagnostic procedures. An insightful commentary in the *British Medical Journal* from 1994 stated the following [6]:

> The view is widely held that experimental methods (randomised controlled trials) are the
> 'gold standard' for evaluation and that observational methods (cohort and case control stud-
> ies) have little or no value. This ignores the limitations of randomised trials, which may
> prove unnecessary, inappropriate, impossible, or inadequate. Many of the problems of con-
> ducting randomised trials could often, in theory, be overcome, but the practical implications
> for researchers and funding bodies mean that this is often not possible. The false conflict

between those who advocate randomised trials in all situations and those who believe observational data provide sufficient evidence needs to be replaced with mutual recognition of the complementary roles of the two approaches. Researchers should be united in their quest for scientific rigour in evaluation, regardless of the method used.

References

1. Proceedings International Society for Geographic Pathology in Stockholm 1937;303–305.
2. Selby JV, Friedman GD, Quesenberry CP Jr, Weiss NS. A case-control study of screening sigmoidoscopy and mortality from colorectal cancer. N Engl J Med 1992 Mar 5;326(10): 653–657.
3. Bull P. What part is played by acute appendicitis in the causation of sterility in young girls and women? Acta Chir Scand 1932;71:155–165.
4. Andersson R, Lambe M, Bergström R. Fertility patterns after appendicectomy: historical cohort study. Br Med J 1999;318(7189):963–967.
5. Statistics from the Swedish Board of Health and Welfare 2006.
6. Black N. Experimental and observational methods of evaluation. Br Med J 1994; 309(6953):540.

Part III
Sources of Error

Chapter 16
Confounding and Bias

In Part II we described how to estimate a measure of association between an exposure and an end point, often a disease. We are interested in "effects" but are only able to measure associations, and we have several procedures to go through before associations can be called "effects." Measures of association emerge for all possible reasons and only some of these relate to "effects." *Effect* is a causal word to be used with care.

It is difficult (in reality impossible) to avoid errors in large-scale population-based studies. It is especially difficult if you have not made it very clear what you want to study and which questions you want to answer. The hypotheses should be the guiding factor in designing the study and in deciding which data you need to collect. The hypotheses are also key when sources of error are discussed and when you plan how best to avoid them. If possible you can present your hypothesis in the form of a diagram, for example a DAG. In this chapter we will consider research based on deduction. A hypothesis is put forward, data are collected to evaluate this hypothesis, and a conclusion is reached. A growing body of literature is, however, based on inductive inference. A large amount of data is collected without a specific hypothesis and data are analyzed to find patterns in the data structure. These studies often rely on powerful computer facilities and laboratory facilities without much biological insight. "Brutal force and ignorance" may describe the new way of analyzing data. It may violate established scientific principles but sometimes produces interesting results.

In this section of the book we will restrict our discussion to deductive studies where the intended study design was valid. This will limit sources of error to factors that can usually be classified as confounding, selection bias, or information bias. Most problems can be described under these headings, but as a reader you should be aware that different terminologies are used to describe and classify sources of error. We will therefore focus upon when and why they occur and how they cause bias. There is no limit to the number of mistakes that you can make in the design phase of a study, and novel designs have to be carefully scrutinized by professional epidemiologists and statisticians. We will leave discussions on this to the scientific literature. We mainly consider sources of error that occur when a valid design meets real-world problems.

J. Olsen et al., *An Introduction to Epidemiology for Health Professionals*,
Springer Series on Epidemiology and Health 1, DOI 10.1007/978-1-4419-1497-2_16,
© Springer Science+Business Media, LLC 2010

First, we should define *bias*, and the authorized definition [1] states

> Deviation of results or inferences from the truth, or processes lead to such deviation. Any trend in the collection, analysis, interpretation, publication, or review of data that can lead to conclusions that are systematically different from the truth.

A study is biased if it produces results that deviate from the truth due to method problems at any stage of research.

Some will use the term bias to include *confounding* – causes of the disease under study that correlate with the exposure of interest. The dictionary's definition includes confounding. Others will say the confounding is not an error but related to the fact that diseases have many causes. Heavy alcohol drinkers do have a higher risk of lung cancer. Probably not because they drink a lot, but because they often tend to smoke. In any case, they have a high lung cancer risk. It is only wrong if we attribute this to their drinking habits because then we may have identified the wrong exposure. We say that the drinking exposure is confounded by its association with smoking habits. If they want to reduce their lung cancer risk they should stop smoking.

Most of the measurements we make are subject to error. Recording a life time history of dietary habits or use of mobile phones during the last 20 years based upon a single recording is of course more error prone than recording of age or sex. Diagnosing a disease may be easy if the disease shows clear symptoms, like measles or bone fractures. It is more difficult to make a subtle diagnosis like attention-deficit hyperactive disorder (ADHD) or to diagnose a slow growing cancer like mycosis fungoides. If we let a number of experts diagnose the same patients they will not always agree, even if they have access to exactly the same information. This information problem will in most cases be a source of bias we need to take into consideration when designing the study. Usually, we will try to design our study in a way that will allow us to know the direction of bias, perhaps even its magnitude. Many of the weak associations we find are probably weak because exposure assessment is too crude or too imprecise or our outcome measures are too unspecific. With better data the strength of the association may be more precisely estimated at a proper larger value.

We design our studies in the hope that those who are invited to take part in the study will accept the invitation, but this is seldom the case. Not all will respond, and those who do will not always remain in the study. This selection into or out of the study group may bias our results. It is well known among those who do surveys in order to get a representative sample of the source population that non-responders will often make the study non-representative. If you want to estimate how many will vote for a given political party, this prediction will be wrong when it is only based on those who responded, and it is a standard practice to adjust for non-responding by using all available information on the non-responders to guess how they would have responded.

In analytical epidemiology we are rarely interested in surveys or representative samples. Surveys provide data for descriptive epidemiology. We are usually interested in identifying determinants of diseases or in evaluating treatments or preventive measures of diseases. Our concern is primarily devoted to how comparable the populations are, or can be made to be, when we make inference about the determinants we study. We call that the *internal validity* of the study and we have a set of guidelines for evaluating this internal validity. We are of course also interested in knowing if this information can be applied to other populations or future patients and not only to the population used for sampling. We have no specific guidelines for estimating this *external validity*. This is an area left for common sense and future experience. The paradox is that we may have ways of calculating confidence limits for the population we used for our study, but once the study is done our interest shifts to other populations. This practice only makes sense if we believe that the causal mechanisms are not time or population specific.

If you read papers on occupational epidemiology you will find terms like *the healthy worker effect*. The term stems from situations where mortality in specific occupations is compared with the mortality of the entire population. These workers will often have a lower than average mortality, which is not surprising. To maintain a full-time physically demanding job, like being a bricklayer or a carpenter, requires good health. It is not a job for those with serious physical handicaps, so the comparison is biased. The comparison group, all in the population, does not produce the expected mortality for workers we study had they not had the occupational exposures. It is thus a type of selection bias that is within the design sphere and thus outside the sources of error we describe in this chapter. We will start with confounding and present problems that are pertinent even in well-designed studies.

Reference

1. Last JM (ed.). A Dictionary of Epidemiology, 3rd Edition. Oxford University Press, New York, 1995.

Chapter 17
Confounding

A *confounder* is an exposure, external to our hypothesis, that biases our measure of association unless it is controlled. When we compare our exposed population with the unexposed comparison group the disease outcome will be different in the two groups even if the exposed had not been exposed. The comparison is confounded by an external factor that has to be a cause of the disease or a correlate for a cause of the disease. It has to be associated with the exposure under study without being in the causal pathway between the exposure and the disease. For a schematic presentation of a simple alternative causal link between E and D (E–C–D), see Fig. 17.1.

Fig. 17.1 Exposure (E), disease (D), and confounder (C)

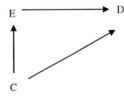

If E is alcohol, D is lung cancer, and C is smoking, smoking would in many situations confound the association E → D. Alcohol intake may be causally related to smoking (probably in a more complicated way than Fig. 17.1 illustrates) and smoking is not part of the causal pathway we take an interest in. Smoking and alcohol are expected to be associated because they may share common causes such as personality, peer pressure, and a genetic predisposition for addiction. In Fig. 17.1 the E–C–D link presents a "back-door" path between E and D.

If E is saturated fat, D is cardiovascular diseases, and C is cholesterol, then C, or at least part of C, is not a confounder but a part of the causal path we take an interest in (it is not just a back-door path between E and D). And the causal diagram would be

J. Olsen et al., *An Introduction to Epidemiology for Health Professionals*,
Springer Series on Epidemiology and Health 1, DOI 10.1007/978-1-4419-1497-2_17,
© Springer Science+Business Media, LLC 2010

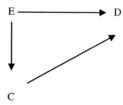

Notice also that the association between E and C is usually not a simple bivariate association but an association present after adjustment for other potential confounders. We thus take an interest in the conditional association between E and C upon adjustment for other confounders. If we have data on both cigarette smoking and inhalation they need not both confound. If all cigarette smokers inhale it is sufficient to adjust for smoking alone.

Table 17.1 shows strong (unusual) confounding (and effect measure modification) by sex. The female sex is a strong determinant of D, and women are much less frequently exposed to E than men (E is an occupational exposure). We can illustrate the association between sex and disease by stratifying our data on exposure as done in Table 17.2.

Table 17.1 A case–control study on the association between hexachlorobenzene exposure (E) and thyroid disease (D), stratified by sex [1]

Stratification on sex	E	D	Controls	OR
Total	+	8	472	
	–	43	1,313	0.52
Men	+	4	422	
	–	1	371	3.52
Women	+	4	50	
	–	42	942	1.79

E = exposure, D = disease.

Table 17.2 Data in Table 17.1 stratified on exposure

Exposure	Sex	D	Controls	OR
Total	M	5	793	
	F	46	992	0.14
+	M	4	422	
	F	4	50	0.12
–	M	1	371	
	F	42	942	0.06

You will rarely see confounding that changes the direction of the exposure–disease association (Table 17.1). When it happens it represents what is called *Simpson's Paradox*. Usually, confounding will attenuate or exaggerate the association (sometimes called negative and positive confounding). A change in the direction of the association is unusual but possible (as in this case and in the comparison between mortality rates in Denmark and Greenland, p. 19).

As illustrated in Fig. 17.1, we avoid confounding by eliminating the association between E and C. The simplest way of eliminating this association is to restrict the study to a limited segment of the population that has only one category of C. If C is age we can restrict the study to a narrow age ban. If C is sex we can restrict the study to males or females. If C is smoking we can perform the study among smokers and non-smokers only. We can also design the study in such a way that no association exists between E and C. The random allocation of E in the randomized trial will usually have this effect. Since exposure is allocated randomly we would expect, at least in a large trial, that the potential confounders (the determinants of the disease we study) will be equally distributed among exposed and unexposed. We can match the follow-up study to make exposed and unexposed comparable concerning the distribution of sex, age, smoking, etc., or we can control for confounding in the analyses, given we have data on confounders, for example by stratifying the analyses as in Table 17.1 or 17.2. Only the randomized trial will, however, adjust for unknown confounders with some degree of certainty, a degree that is reflected in the confidence interval.

In non-experimental studies we try to capture some of these unknown confounders by adjusting (deconfounding) for variables that correlate with many conditions, like sex, age, or socioeconomic status.

Confounding is a potential problem that receives much attention in most epidemiological studies, but it is not equally serious in all studies. If you study the association between use of a specific component in soap and hand eczema there may not be many correlates of this exposure that are causally linked to hand eczema unless they are in the soap you study. If you study effects of treatment, your comparison between treated and untreated patients may be strongly confounded by the severity of the disease (*confounding by indication* for the treatment). Assuming this comparison is not based upon a randomization of the treatment, the two patient groups are not expected to be comparable. Doctors are trained to select the best possible treatment given the state of the disease, and if they succeed in selecting the proper candidates for treatment treated patients will not be comparable with non-treated patients. There were reasons for using this treatment for these specific patients, an indication for the treatment (confounding by indication). This type of confounding is a main reason for the need to study treatment effects in randomized trials. Good clinical decision making tends to ruin our options for studying treatment effects in non-randomized studies, and the better the clinicians are the more they will confound our source population "by their valid indications for treatment."

If we take an interest in a specific dietary component and its possible health effects, this dietary component will usually be closely linked to other dietary components. Say you take an interest in beta-carotene and its effect on lung cancer. Beta-carotene in food comes in a package, like in a carrot, and beta-carotene is just one of many components in the carrot. Therefore, eating carrots correlates with other food components. Furthermore, people who eat carrots usually also eat other types of vegetables. Add to this that eating carrots replaces other types of food items. Adjusting for all these factors may well be impossible in a non-randomized trial. Studies have shown that eating a diet rich in beta-carotene is associated with low lung cancer risks, but this association has not been found in randomized trials where beta-carotene was allocated by randomization. The reason could be that the protective effect of eating carrots was not caused by beta-carotene (ecological fallacy) or that beta-carotene only has protective effects in combination with what else is in the carrot. It is also possible, but not likely, that the randomized trials got it all wrong which could happen if the exposure time was too short.

The use of *matching* in the follow-up study is a straightforward and conceptually simple technique. In individual matching on, say, smoking you select an unexposed with the same smoking history as your selected exposed (individual matching). In frequency matching you sample unexposed so they have the same smoking frequencies as you have in the population of exposed. Using matching in a case–control study is quite different. Matching in a case–control study does not in itself solve the problem of confounding. The reason is that when you match cases with controls you change the confounder distribution among cases to make it similar to the confounder distribution in controls (not similar among exposed and unexposed). If the exposure is a cause of the disease you introduce confounding even if there was no confounding in the source population. If both the exposure and the confounders are causally linked to the disease they will be associated when you stratify or match on case status since it is a collider. If you use the terminology used in DAGs you will see that E and C become associated when you stratify on D (match on D) since D is a collider in this diagram:

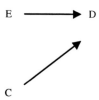

E and C are not associated in the population. There is no arrow from C to E.

In a stratified analysis with no adjustment, except the adjustment that is part of the matched design, you have to count how many matched sets you have that follow the pattern indicated in Table 17.3 (matched sets with one case and one control).

Table 17.3 A matched case–control study

Exposure		
Type	Case	Control
1	0	0
2	+	0
3	0	+
4	+	+

$+$ = exposure, 0 = no exposure.

The matched sets of types 1 and 4 provide no indication of a causal association. In all these sets neither the case nor the control is exposed [1] or they are both exposed [2]. All information is given in type 2 sets (indicating a positive association between exposure and disease) and type 3 sets (indicating a negative, protective, effect of the exposure). Our measure of association will simply be type 2 sets divided by type 3 sets.

Any study result can always be claimed to be confounded and most study results are probably confounded to some extent. Still, it should be realized that confounding needs to be strong to explain away strong associations with a high risk ratio for the disease.

Table 17.4 [2] shows the expected confounding effect by smoking if smoking is not adjusted for. The comparison group has the smoking prevalence shown in the table (Exp–), and all the Exp+ groups represent different levels of confounding by smoking among the exposed and assuming no effect of the exposure. In this table, smoking is considered a strong risk factor with relative risks of 10 and 20. The deviations of the RR away from 1.00 are explained entirely by confounding by smoking. As seen, smoking prevalences have to deviate substantially between the compared groups to explain relative risks lower than 0.6 or higher than 1.5. Confounding by smoking cannot, under the given assumptions, explain an RR lower than 0.15 or higher than 3.08, even when no one or all smoke in the exposed group.

Table 17.4 How much confounding could smoking cause?

Exp	Non-smokers (1x)	Smokers (10x)	Heavy smokers (20x)	RR
+	100	–	–	0.15
+	80	20	–	0.43
+	70	30	–	0.57
+	60	35	5	0.78
–	50	40	10	1.00
+	40	45	15	1.22
+	30	50	20	1.43
+	20	55	25	1.65
+	10	60	30	1.86
+	–	65	35	2.08
+	–	25	75	2.69
+	–	–	100	3.08

References

1. Sala M, Sunyer J, Herrero C, To-Figueras J, Grimalt J. Association between serum concentrations of hexachlorobenzene and polychlorobiphenyls with thyroid hormone and liver enzymes in a sample of the general population. Occup Environ Med 2001;58(3):172–177.
2. Axelson O. Confounding by smoking in occupational epidemiology. Br J Ind Med 1989;46:505–507.

Chapter 18
Information Bias

Most studies are based on data that are recorded with some errors. We may be able to record gender precisely, birth weight with some errors, birth length with more errors, past occupational exposures with even more uncertainties, not to mention long-term dietary habits or use of mobile phones years ago. Sometimes diseases are diagnosed by their symptoms only, like depression. Sometimes there may be objective signs, as for hypertension. In clinical practice, there will often be some disagreement between groups of clinical experts when making diagnoses. In a study we may have errors in our measurement of exposures, endpoints, and/or confounders. If these errors lead to bias (they normally will) we call this type of bias *information bias*. If our measurement is a categorical variable, such as a diagnostic code or a code for gender, we talk about misclassification or *misclassification bias*.

In large studies we often either have to rely on existing data or have to make clinical tests that cannot be too invasive and often have to be inexpensive with the limited research funds available in most countries. By comparing how a given test performs on known cases and known non-cases diagnosed with better clinical tests (golden standard) we can quantify the amount of misclassification we may expect in the study by estimating sensitivity and specificity (Table 18.1).

Table 18.1 Applying a study test to known cases and known non-cases

	Known disease status	
Study test	Cases	Non-cases
Positive	*a*	*b*
Negative	*c*	*d*
Total	*a+c*	*b+d*

The proportion of all diseased classified as test positives (cases) in the study by the study test is a/(a+c). This is an estimate of the *sensitivity* of the test, the probability of being test positive given the tested have the disease ($P(\text{test+}|\text{disease})$).

The proportion of truly non-diseased we expect to classify as such in the study using the study test will be d/(b+d). This measure is an estimate of the *specificity* of the test, the probability of being classified as test negative given the tested do not

J. Olsen et al., *An Introduction to Epidemiology for Health Professionals*,
Springer Series on Epidemiology and Health 1, DOI 10.1007/978-1-4419-1497-2_18,
© Springer Science+Business Media, LLC 2010

have the disease (P(test–|no disease)). These estimates of sensitivity and specificity come with some uncertainties based on who takes part in the study, which test is used, and the sample size.

If, on the other hand, we want to estimate the probability that a positive test identifies a diseased we need to know the prevalence of the disease in that population, P. Given this information we can construct the probabilities of falling into the table's four cells, and these four probabilities are presented in Table 18.2.

Table 18.2 Probability distribution for test positives and test negatives according to disease occurrence

Test	Cases	Non-cases	All
Positive	$P \times$ sens	$(1 - P)(1 - $spec$)$	$\hat{P}$
Negative	$P \times (1 - $sens$)$	$(1 - P)$spec	$1 - \hat{P}$
All	P	$1 - P$	

Sens = sensitivity; Spec = specificity; P = prevalence proportion of having the disease; $\hat{P}$ = prevalence proportion of being test positive.

From Table 18.2 it is seen that the estimated prevalence $\hat{P}$ is a function of the true prevalence, P, and the sensitivity and specificity of the test [1]:

$$\hat{P} = P \times \text{sens} + (1 - P)(1 - \text{spec})$$

$$\hat{P} = P \times \text{sens} + 1 - \text{spec} - P + P\text{spec}$$

$$\hat{P} = 1 - \text{spec} + P(\text{sens} + \text{spec} - 1)$$

$$P = \frac{\hat{P} + \text{spec} - 1}{\text{sens} + \text{spec} - 1}$$

Given the information on sensitivity and specificity and the proportion of test positives we can estimate the "true" prevalence if we want to quantify the amount of bias caused by misclassification of the diseased by using an imperfect diagnostic instrument.

Assume we have a study with complete follow-up and with no misclassification as in Table 18.3.

Table 18.3 Follow-up study with no disease misclassification

Exp	N	D	RR
Yes	1,000	200	
No	1,000	100	$\frac{200/1,000}{100/1,000} = 2.0$

Table 18.4 Follow-up study with some misclassification of the disease status

Exp	N	D	RR
Yes	1,000	160(200 × 0.80)	
No	1,000	80(100 × 0.80)	$\frac{160/1,000}{80/1,000} = 2.0$

If we now use a test to identify the diseased that has a sensitivity of 0.80 and a specificity of 1.00 we could expect to get as in Table 18.4.

Notice that a relative measure of association is not biased by a low sensitivity in this example as long as the sensitivity is the same in the groups to be compared.

Assume now that the sensitivity is 1.0 and the specificity is 0.90; if so we get Table 18.5.

Table 18.5 Follow-up study with misclassification of the disease status

Exp	N	D	RR
Yes	1,000	200 + 80 (800 × 0.10)	
No	1,000	100 + 90 (900 × 0.10)	$\frac{280/1,000}{190/1,000} = 1.47$

Since sensitivity and specificity are the same for exposed and unexposed we say the misclassification is non-differential (*non-differential misclassification*) and as seen in this example this type of misclassification will offer bias-relative effect estimates toward 1. A general rule, as illustrated in this simple example, is that ratio measures are less sensitive to low values of sensitivity than low values of specificity. That need not be the case for absolute measures of association. The risk difference in Table 18.3 is (200/1,000 – 100/1,000) = 0.10. In Table 18.4 we get (160/1,000 – 80/1,000) = 0.08. And in Table 18.5 (280/1,000 – 190/1,000) = 0.09.

If the misclassification is differential (*differential misclassification*), the sensitivity and/or specificity differ(s) among exposed and unexposed and bias can be in any direction.

You will often find statements in scientific papers saying that since misclassification of either exposure data or disease data was non-differential the measure of association was attenuated (relative effect measures closer to 1; absolute estimates of effect measures closer to 0). This is often overstating reality. Non-differential misclassification will attenuate the measure of association in most realistic situations for dichotomized exposures and outcomes, but there are usually other sources of bias that may operate in an opposite direction and the net effect may be unknown. Bias related to non-differential misclassification will not always be toward no effect; e.g., if the disease state is wrongly coded (exposed coded 0 and unexposed coded 1 where it should have been the opposite) this will produce non-differential misclassification that biases our measure away from the null – it will in fact reverse the measure of association. If exposures and diseases have more than two categories non-differential misclassification can in some situations bias results away from the null. Misclassification of confounders may bias results in any direction [2].

In a case–control study you often identify cases from a disease register or from medical records. Once the cases have been identified it may be possible to check if they meet the diagnostic criteria you want them to fulfill. In cancer research it is common practice in high-quality case–control studies to let a reference pathologist with known and recognized expertise go through the existing medical records and slides. Only if he/she accepts the documentation for the diagnostic criteria is the patient admitted to the case group. The reason for this quality control is to increase the specificity of the diagnostic procedures and to avoid the potential attenuating of effects by including non-cases in the case group. To see how this works, assume you have a closed population with the following data at the end of follow-up and assume no diagnostic uncertainties (Table 18.6).

Table 18.6 Follow-up study, no misclassification

Exp	N	D	$\bar{D}$
+	1,000	200	800
−	1,000	100	900

D = disease, $\bar{D}$ = no disease.

The relative risk is $2.0 \left(\frac{200/1,000}{100/1,000} \right)$ and if we sample a 1:1 case–cohort study we will get (assuming no sampling variation and that controls reflect the exposure distribution in the source population – 50% exposures) as in Table 18.7.

Table 18.7 Case–cohort sampling from Table 18.6

Exp	Cases	Controls
+	200	150
−	100	150
All	300	300

$$OR = \frac{200/100}{150/150} = 2.0$$

Now assume when we select the case–control study that the diagnosing is based on diagnostic routines that have a sensitivity of 0.80 and a specificity of 0.90. The data in our population would then look like in Table 18.8.

Table 18.8 Follow-up study, misclassification

Exp	N	$\hat{D}$
+	1,000	$(200 \times 0.80) + (800 \times 0.10) = 240$
−	1,000	$(100 \times 0.80) + (900 \times 0.10) = 170$

$RR = \frac{760/1,000}{830/1,000} = 1.41$

A case–cohort sampling would give as in Table 18.9.

Table 18.9 Case–cohort
sampling from Table 18.8

Exp	Cases	Control
+	240	205
–	170	205
All	410	410

$$OR = \frac{240/170}{205/205} = 1.41$$

If our reference pathologist could eliminate the false positive cases, our case–control sampling would give the result as stated in Table 18.10, given no sampling variation.

Table 18.10 Case–cohort
study, sampling from
Table 18.8, no false positives

Exp	Cases	Control
+	160	120
–	80	120
All	240	240

$$OR = \frac{160/80}{120/120} = 2.0$$

and we would obtain an unbiased estimate of RR (2.0).

As a general rule you should try to reduce measurement errors as much as possible and what remains of measurement errors you should try to make non-differential. That can sometimes be achieved by using *blinding*. Make sure diagnosing is made without information on exposure status. When exposures are measured, for example in the laboratory, blind the lab technicians to the disease status and make sure cases and controls are analyzed in randomly balanced sets.

References

1. Olsen J. Screening for karcinogene stoffer i arbejdsmiljøet. Kommentar (In Danish) Ugeskr Læger 1978;140(51):3248–3249.
2. Greenland S. Confounding and misclassification. Am J Epidemiol 1985;122:495–506.

Chapter 19
Selection Bias

The most common type of selection bias in case–control studies and in surveys is caused by non-responders. Not all accept to join the study among those selected as eligible and therefore invited.

Imagine a survey that aims at estimating the prevalence of obesity in the population. Imagine that our random sample of the population (80% responders) shows the results presented in Table 19.1.

Table 19.1 Cross-sectional study on obesity

	N	$\%_1$	$\%_2$	$\%_3$	$\%_4$
Obese	300	30	37.5	50	30
Not obese	500	50	62.5	50	70
Missing	200	20	–	–	–
Total	1,000	100	100	100	100

The second column, $\%_1$, shows the distribution of responders (obese and not obese), and non-responders, $\%_2$, indicates that 37.5% are obese under the assumption of no selection bias (the non-responders also include 37.5% obese). $\%_3$ shows 50% are obese under the assumption that all non-responders are obese, and $\%_4$ indicates 30% are obese under the assumption that no non-responders are obese. We may conclude that between 30 and 50% are obese in this population (maximal selection bias), and if the non-responders cause no selection bias our estimate is 37.5. If we have some information on non-responders we may provide a better estimate of the prevalence of obesity in the population.

In some randomized trials less than 20% accept the invitation to the study, and in time-consuming follow-up studies often less than 50% take part in the study. In case–control studies participation rates for cases may be high but could be low for controls who do not have the same incentive to take part in the study. It is important to realize that the threat to validity caused by selection bias differs between the different study designs. The reason is that for selection to cause bias selection has to be associated with both the exposure and the outcome. Since the outcome will not be known at the time of invitation to the follow-up study it is impossible to decide upon

J. Olsen et al., *An Introduction to Epidemiology for Health Professionals*,
Springer Series on Epidemiology and Health 1, DOI 10.1007/978-1-4419-1497-2_19,
© Springer Science+Business Media, LLC 2010

participation based on information that is not known at the time of recruitment. The decision to take part can only be associated with the outcome, through chance or through other variables (cause confounding). In the case–control study the situation is different. Women who have breast cancer and have used oral contraceptives (OCs) may be interested in taking part in a case–control study that aims at estimating breast cancer risk among OC users. Cancer patients or controls who never used OCs may not have the same incentive to take part in the study.

People invited to an ongoing follow-up study cannot base their acceptance on an unknown disease they may or may not get in the future, so selection bias is less likely and the internal validity need not be influenced by the selection if the study is well controlled for confounding factors. However, selection may well make the participants different from those who declined the invitation to take part in the study and that may often lead to a lower disease risk among the participants. This is expected because people with poor health more often refuse to take part in research for various reasons. We may therefore expect a different set of confounders among participants than among non-participants and we may often see less confounding in the group that participated in the study than among all who were invited. In the randomized trial, selection cannot be related to exposure except by chance. Exposures are distributed according to randomization, and outcomes are unknown at the time of informed consent (and before randomization) but as in an observational study those who participated may have a different disease risk than those who refused. Lack of compliance to the protocol during follow-up can and will, however, often lead to selection bias of the internal comparisons in a randomized trial and in other follow-up studies.

Selection bias in follow-up studies at baseline is mainly related to the external validity or generalization of our study results. The question we have to ask ourselves is whether there are differences between the population from which we have collected our data and the population we want to generalize to, and whether these differences are expected to modify our results. (External validity is a question about effect measure modification.) The internal validity in a randomized trial may be high, but the patients are usually highly selected. Will the treatment work and have the same set of side effects for other patients?

In follow-up studies we often have to accept that participants leave the study before follow-up ends. In many cases, this loss to follow-up may be linked to both the exposure and the disease under study. In a study on exposures to cleaning agents and hand eczema, those with vulnerable skin may change jobs before they get eczema as a response to early markers of eczema. If all susceptible persons are removed from the exposed cohort by this self-selection a naïve analysis of data may show the exposure to be protective. Or imagine a randomized trial for a given pain killer. Those who remain in pain will probably be less likely to continue a treatment that does not work, and compliance is expected to be lower among those who received such treatment. Lack of compliance to the protocol is therefore expected to be more common in the arm of the study that receives the less effective treatment, and lack of compliance can eliminate some (and perhaps most) of the design benefits achieved by the randomization.

Loss to follow-up often increases with follow-up time, and a randomized trial is a less attractive study option if long-term follow-up is needed. Since selection bias during follow-up is not unlikely the "intention to treat analyses" may remain "valid" but almost meaningless. They may provide a valid test of the null hypothesis if the study is powered to provide such a test, but the study provides no useful estimate of effects because the "intention to treat" correlates too little with actual treatment. The randomization is a poor instrumental variable for actual exposure.

Selection into a follow-up study only causes selection bias (it may cause confounding) of the measure of association if the selection is associated with both the exposure and the end point, which is unlikely, but compliance to the follow-up regime becomes very important. Lack of compliance to follow-up may well be associated with both the exposure and the outcome. Most epidemiologists would, on the informed consent form, emphasize the importance of staying in the study if enrolled. The advice to potential participants should in many cases be "if in doubt, stay out."

Selection bias at recruitment is of major concern in descriptive studies and in case–control studies. If a survey aims at estimating the prevalence of ADHD and not all in the random sample participate our estimate will be biased if the prevalence of ADHD differs among the participants and the non-participants, which is likely.

In a case–control study (like in the follow-up study) our aim is to quantify an association between an exposure and a disease. That estimate is subject to selection bias if the selection is associated with both the exposure and the disease. Since both the exposure and the disease may be known at the time of recruitment the decision to accept or reject the invitation can cause selection bias. If the exposure is a genetic variant or a biomarker of an environmental pollutant the participants will usually not have that information when they decide to take part in the study, and such a study is therefore less prone to selection bias.

Assume you want to study the association between the use of oral contraceptives (OC) and breast cancer (BC) and assume that the study would look like the data in Table 19.2 if all participated.

Table 19.2 Case–control study on the use of oral contraception (OC) and breast cancer (BC)

OC use	BC	Controls	OR
+	150	120	
–	250	280	
All	400	400	$OR = \frac{150/250}{120/280} = 1.40$

In most situations not all 800 will accept taking part in the interviewing. An 80% participation rate may be considered good and 50% poor, although there are no well-accepted cut-off points since the potential bias factor depends on many other factors.

Selection bias is likely because not everybody has the same incentive to participate. Women with breast cancer may find the hypothesis interesting if they have used OCs, whereas breast cancer women who never used OCs may find it a waste of time to take part in the study. Controls participate mainly for altruistic reasons, and we could end up with case–control data like those presented in Table 19.3.

Table 19.3 Participants in the case–control study

OC use	BC	Controls	OR
+	135	96	
–	185	224	
All	320	320	$OR = \frac{135/185}{96/224} = 1.70$

Notice that we have 20% non-participants for both cases and controls and our OR is biased toward a stronger association (from 1.40 to 1.70). The reason is that the selection is related to both the exposure and the disease as seen in Table 19.4 where exposure- and disease-specific participation percentages are displayed.

Table 19.4 Participants in the case–control study presented in percent of all in each of the four exposure–disease cells

OC use	BC (%)	Controls (%)
+	90	80
–	74	80
All	80	80

It can be shown [1] that in some situations

$$OR_{biased} = OR_{true} \times OR_{participation\ rates}$$
$$1.70 = 1.40 \times \frac{90/74}{80/80}$$

The risk of selection bias can be reduced if it is acceptable to keep the detailed hypothesis unknown to the participants. Many case–control studies address a whole series of hypotheses at the same time, and it should be acceptable on the consent form to state, for example, that the study is on lifestyle factors and drug use as possible risk factors of breast cancer, without further details. In genetic studies involving the screening of hundreds of thousands of genes, requesting specific informed consent is not even an option.

If the case–control study is nested within a well-described cohort it may be possible to obtain information on the combined distribution of exposures and outcomes among the non-responders. In other situations it is advisable to get at least some information from part of the non-responders. A sample of non-responders may be willing to provide some data to the study although they did not accept to provide all the information. The information you would like to have the most is information on exposure.

Reference

1. Greenland S. Response and follow-up bias in cohort studies. Am J Epidemiol 1977;106: 184–187.

Chapter 20
Making Inference and Making Decisions

The designs described in Chapter 2 allow you to estimate associations between the exposures under study and the corresponding health outcome. Making *causal inference* is a more complicated issue. No design and no statistical procedures will in themselves allow you to make causal inference. You can only be more or less certain about causal relations, and making causal inference rests to some extent on subjective consideration. However, the opinion of those who know the subject matter well carries more weight than the opinion of ignorants, although the latter could be right. History shows that the skillful more often got it right, because knowledge allows you to identify some non-causal associations. Skills will allow you to put hypotheses to critical tests that often will reveal associations caused by bias or confounding.

Epidemiologists use terms like *risk indicators* to describe simple statistical associations that need not be causal. Being unmarried is a risk indicator of getting cancer of the cervix, but marital status has no direct causal link to the disease. A *risk factor* is a stronger term, used when we think the association could be causal but we do not really know. We may, for example, say that having frequent sex with several partners is a risk factor for cancer of the cervix, although we do not think that sex in itself is a risk factor. Still, we believe that if women reduce their number of sex partners they reduce their risk of cervical cancer because having sex occasionally carries a risk. We now have enough information to classify certain types of human papiloma virus transmitted by the sexual act as carcinogens because the cumulative documentation for a causal effect is overwhelming. Still, causal terms are to be used cautiously. Terms like etiologic fractions or attributable fractions should not be used unless we think we have a causal relation. Causal conclusions usually require substantial convincing evidence from several studies.

Some hold the naïve belief that a randomized trial will provide evidence that allows you to make causal inference, but most randomized trials have shortcomings, and even a perfect design will produce a conclusion based on statistical significance testing that will be wrong 5% of the time if the exposure has no effect, if the null hypothesis is true.

Making causal inference in public health and clinical practice is related to the decision to act since there are no reasons to act on non-causal associations. Many elements go into this decision process. First of all, we have to take into consideration

J. Olsen et al., *An Introduction to Epidemiology for Health Professionals*,
Springer Series on Epidemiology and Health 1, DOI 10.1007/978-1-4419-1497-2_20,
© Springer Science+Business Media, LLC 2010

the consequences of acting on a given epidemiologic result and weigh that against the consequences of not acting. If we, for example, find that drinking eight cups of coffee per day or more during pregnancy correlates with behavioral problems in the offspring during childhood we may decide to warn pregnant women against such heavy coffee consumption, although we may be far from certain that the association is causal. We are quite certain that drinking no coffee or drinking smaller amounts of coffee during pregnancy will cause no harm (except perhaps to the coffee producer). If we find that eating fish or sea animals during pregnancy in the Faroe Islands may impair brain function in the offspring, the decision process may be more difficult. If the association is strong we should warn against eating this type of food. If the association is weak the decision to act is more difficult. Replacing an exposure with another may carry other health hazards and the intervention may have undesirable cultural and economic consequences. The population should of course be informed about our findings because the final decision to act upon the results is in their hands.

Using a precautionary principle, or giving people the benefit of the doubt, may not always be as simple as it sounds. There are some indications that the use of mobile phones causes health problems. Should we warn people against using these phones? We know that human life existed before the phones were invented although it may be hard for some to comprehend. They may carry risks when driving while talking on a mobile phone, but, on the other hand, the phones have uses that increase quality of life for many and they may even be used to prevent health hazards or to get help if help is needed.

In deciding when to act, causal inference is key since the causality is a necessary condition for prevention to work; at least that prevention will lead to changes that include a causal link. If we reduce the number of sexual partners we reduce the risk of HIV and cancer of the cervix because the action will eliminate some causal links. If we had an effective vaccination program that could eliminate the causal link between the virus and cancer then the behavioral changes would not be needed to reduce the cancer risk but may be needed for other reasons.

B. Hill's causal criteria [1] state what speaks in favor of a causal effect, although none of them prove causality, either taken in isolation or in combination. In fact, Hill never used the term criteria but preferred to talk about considerations or guidelines. Whether criteria or guidelines, they are as follows:

1. *Strength of association*: The stronger the association, the more likely the association represents causality. Most will agree that strong associations are less likely caused by confounding than weak associations and are therefore causal candidates, but strength of association provides no guarantees. Strong associations may be a result of bias and confounding, especially in situations where the exposure is part of a combined set of exposures, like when you study nicotine that comes together with hundreds of chemicals in tobacco smoke, caffeine that is part of coffee, or beta-carotene that is part of certain vegetables. All these "exposures" correlate strongly with all other exposures in the combined package that "carries" the potential "cause." For a confounder to explain the association it would need to be associated with the exposures and to be causally linked to the

outcome. Notice that in the theory of component causes the strength of an association is a function of the prevalence of the other component causes in the causal field, leading to the disease. Obesity is a strong risk factor for diabetes in populations with a high genetic susceptibility to diabetes if these genetic factors are in the same causal field as obesity. In a population with a lower prevalence of these genetic factors the risk associated with obesity is expected to be lower.

2. *Consistency*: Consistency means that the association can be replicated. The idea is that a chance finding will usually not be replicated. The search for genetic causes of diseases has provided many associations that could not be replicated. That is not unexpected if the prior belief is limited and many associations are examined.

3. *Specificity*: A given exposure should have a specific effect according to this criterion. Experience shows, however, that many exposures have several health effects and there are often no biological reasons to expect only one. If an exposure during organogenesis leads to a specific malformation, like cleft lip, it may, however, raise more concern than if the exposure is related to all types of malformations. In the latter case, we will be more concerned about sources of bias related to the diagnosing of malformations or the selection of people to the study.

4. *Temporality*: This may be the only criterion that all would request to be fulfilled, that the cause precedes the effect. Notice that this criterion is difficult to document. Many diseases develop over long preclinical time spans and they could in this time period impact exposures like dietary factors.

5. *Biological gradient*: This refers to a dose–response or dose–effect relation; that an increasing dose leads to an increasing incidence of the disease. It is expected that an increasing cumulative dose leads to an increasing cumulative incidence based on the causal fields theory. The more times you cross a street, the more likely it is that at some point in time you will be hit by a car (that all the component causes that lead to an accident will be present). How an increasing intensity of exposure leads to a higher risk is more difficult to understand unless it is related to an increasing probability of the exposure to reach the target organ. The dose–response relation may reflect an increasing number of de facto exposed at higher exposure levels.

6. *Plausibility*: If we understand how a given exposure causes a disease we tend to believe a causal explanation more than if we have no mechanistic explanation. A biological/sociological theory will also make it easier to make testable predictions that can be falsified. But remember that X-rays or tobacco smoke also caused cancer before we knew the mechanism behind this association.

7. *Coherence*: This criterion is linked to the criteria of plausibility and consistency.

8. *Experimental evidence*: If our results are supported by findings based on carefully controlled experiments in humans (or in animals) it speaks in favor of a causal inference.

9. *Analogy*: If the association we see has been found for other similar exposures it speaks in favor of causation. Many believe that passive smoking causes lung cancer because the findings fit well with what we would expect from our studies on active smoking and our dose–response estimates.

Most experts will use all or some of these criteria when they are to summarize results and make causal inference. None of these criteria, if fulfilled, will prove causality taken individually or together. Such proof does not exist. Notice that criteria 1, 2, and 5 deal directly with the empirical associations (epistemologic criteria). Criteria 3, 4, 6, 7, and 9 have to do with the causality itself (ontologic criteria).

Since we will never be able to prove causality we need to take action without such proof. In order to do that we often need to quantify the probability of the association to be causal. *The International Agency for Research on Cancer (IARC)* classifies possible carcinogenic exposures using different categories. Notice that they use strong causal language – stronger than what we recommend – probably to advocate action where they believe action is justified. The following text is taken from the IARC guidelines [2]:

"Group 1 – The agent (mixture) is carcinogenic to humans.

The exposure circumstance entails exposures that are carcinogenic to humans.

This category is used when there is *sufficient evidence* of carcinogenicity in humans. Exceptionally, an agent (mixture) may be placed in this category when evidence of carcinogenicity in humans is less than sufficient but there is *sufficient evidence* of carcinogenicity in experimental animals and strong evidence in exposed humans that the agent (mixture) acts through a relevant mechanism of carcinogenicity.

Group 2

This category includes agents, mixtures and exposure circumstances for which, at one extreme, the degree of evidence of carcinogenicity in humans is almost sufficient, as well as those for which, at the other extreme, there are no human data but for which there is evidence of carcinogenicity in experimental animals. Agents, mixtures and exposure circumstances are assigned to either group 2A (probably carcinogenic to humans) or group 2B (possibly carcinogenic to humans) on the basis of epidemiological and experimental evidence of carcinogenicity and other relevant data.

Group 2A – The agent (mixture) is probably carcinogenic to humans.

The exposure circumstance entails exposures that are probably carcinogenic to humans.

This category is used when there is *limited evidence* of carcinogenicity in humans and *sufficient evidence* of carcinogenicity in experimental animals and strong evidence that the carcinogenesis is mediated by a mechanism that also operates in humans. Exceptionally, an agent, mixture or exposure circumstance may be classified in this category solely on the basis of *limited evidence* of carcinogenicity in humans.

Group 2B – The agent (mixture) is possibly carcinogenic to humans.

The exposure circumstance entails exposures that are possibly carcinogenic to humans.

This category is used for agents, mixtures and exposure circumstances for which there is *limited evidence* of carcinogenicity in humans and less than *sufficient evidence* of carcinogenicity in experimental animals. It may also be used when there is *inadequate evidence* of carcinogenicity in humans but there is *sufficient evidence* of carcinogenicity in experimental animals. In some instances, an agent, mixture or exposure circumstance for which there is *inadequate evidence* of carcinogenicity in humans but *limited evidence* of carcinogenicity in experimental animals together with supporting evidence from other relevant data may be placed in this group.

Group 3 – The agent (mixture or exposure circumstance) is not classifiable as to its carcinogenicity to humans.

This category is used most commonly for agents, mixtures and exposure circumstances for which the *evidence of carcinogenicity* is *inadequate* in humans and *inadequate* or *limited* in experimental animals. Exceptionally, agents (mixtures) for which the *evidence of carcinogenicity* is *inadequate* in humans but *sufficient* in experimental animals may be placed in this category when there is strong evidence that the mechanism of carcinogenicity in experimental animals does not operate in humans.

Agents, mixtures and exposure circumstances that do not fall into any other group are also placed in this category.

Group 4 – The agent (mixture) is probably not carcinogenic to humans.

This category is used for agents or mixtures for which there is *evidence suggesting lack of carcinogenicity* in humans and in experimental animals. In some instances, agents or mixtures for which there is *inadequate evidence* of carcinogenicity in humans but *evidence suggesting lack of carcinogenicity* in experimental animals, consistently and strongly supported by a broad range of other relevant data, may be classified in this group" [3].

These guidelines illustrate that causal inference has strong subjective elements; words like sufficient, inadequate, limited will not be understood in the same way by everybody, and experts will continue to disagree about the probability that a given association reflects causality. Expert reviews or meta-analyses may reduce the disagreement but will not eliminate it and may make it more transparent what the disagreements are about.

References

1. Hill AB. The environment and disease: association or causation? Proc R Soc Med 1965;58:295–300.
2. http://www.iarc.fr/
3. WHO, IARC. IARC Monographs on the Evaluation of Carcinogenic Risks to Humans, Volume 78, Ionizing Radiation, Part 2: Some Internally Deposited Radionuclides. IARC Press, Lyon, France, 2001.

Chapter 21
Sources of Error in Public Health Epidemiology

The public health worker will need to have more detailed knowledge of sources of bias since he/she will mainly work with non-experimental data and will have to make decisions that may impact the health of many people in both positive and negative ways.

Most study results are presented with a confidence interval (or confidence limits) around a measure of association, but the calculations are done under assumptions that will almost never be true, and confidence limits do not provide a true range of uncertainty (or confidence) of the study result we need to take into consideration.

A true set of confidence limits should take uncontrolled confounding, selection bias, and misclassification into consideration. The public health worker often needs to be able to perform sensitivity analyses to address questions of the type "How much uncontrolled confounding is needed to explain away a given association?" or "How much differential misclassification or selection bias is needed to produce the effect estimates we obtained?" Some of the simple techniques provided in this book can be used to address questions of this type. More advanced methods often require more detailed information and access to sophisticated software.

Although most sources of error can be assigned to one of the types of bias and confounding described in the chapter there are errors that fall outside these classes of bias categories.

Regression toward the mean is one such "error" that should be known to people working in public health and clinical epidemiology. The "error" describes the tendency for extreme values to regress toward the mean when measurements are repeated. Assume you measure blood pressure (BP) in a population and get this distribution (Fig. 21.1).

If you select all those with a blood pressure above x and put them on a diet low in salt and measure their blood pressure later you will most likely find their blood pressure to be lower at the second reading, even if nobody followed your dietary advice. A proportion of those selected from the extreme parts of the distribution will regress toward the mean. The reason is that your measure of blood pressure, $\widehat{BP}$, is a function of the true blood pressure (BP) plus a measurement error (could be biological variations and random variation related to the measuring itself), ε, so

Fig. 21.1 The distribution of blood pressure (BP) in the population

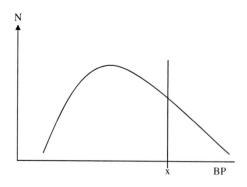

$$\widehat{BP} = BP + \varepsilon$$

These errors could be negative or positive, large and small, but according to the theory of random measurement errors they will for all measurements sum up to 0; $\Sigma\varepsilon = 0$ for the entire population. When we select from extreme parts of the distribution we oversample those with high (or low) measurement errors. When we select from the extreme we take a biased sample and our sum of ε will be larger than 0 from the high end of the distribution and below 0 from the low end. The reason is that our measure of blood pressure, $\widehat{BP}$, may be high because BP was high or because ε was high, or both, and on average $\Sigma\varepsilon$ will be > 0. When the participants return for new blood pressure measurements these new measures will, according to the rule of measurement errors, again sum up to 0. Their new blood pressure measurements regress toward the mean of the distribution and the magnitude of the regression will depend on the size of the measurement errors. Notice that the measure regresses *toward* the mean, not *to* the mean.

This simple error is often found in naïve analyses of new interventions or treatments done by amateurs, but it is unfortunately also seen in more serious studies from time to time, and it is important to remember that the problem comes in different disguises.

When lithium was first introduced as a drug to prevent bipolar disorders, the case series showed the following typical pattern of changes in mood after being treated with lithium as illustrated in Fig. 21.2.

The critique that followed the publication [1] pointed out that the association could reflect regression toward the mean. If you start treatment when patients have the highest level of variance in mood, they can only regress toward less variation. Subsequent analyses did, however, show that the association was real. The treated patients had a long history of large mood changes over long time periods before they were treated with lithium.

If you do a study where the aim is to identify "predictors" of a disease, say, cytokines related to preterm labor, your predictions will be overstated in your study due to regression toward the mean. Part of your measure of the association is related

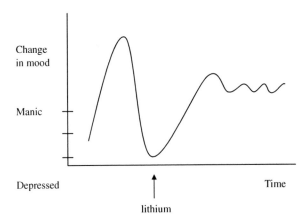

Fig. 21.2 Mood variation before and after treatment with lithium

to chance and a new study with a different data source will most likely show lower predictive values. The associations will regress toward no association.

Berkson Bias

The public health epidemiologist should also be familiar with *Berkson bias* (*or Berksonian bias*) because this type of bias may also come in different disguises [2].

Berkson demonstrated how different medical conditions could be associated among hospital patients although they were not associated in the population. He noted that clinicians had the impression that cholecystitis was associated with diabetes and the gallbladder was often removed as part of diabetes treatment for that reason. How could such an idea come about even if the two diseases are not associated in the population?

How this association is generated in hospital patients can be found in Berkson's original paper [2]. We will demonstrate that people who have two diseases (or more), for example diabetes and cholecystitis, are more likely to be hospitalized than those with only one of the diseases. The idea is simply that you can be hospitalized either for one disease or for the other. Both diseases provide a cue for hospitalization.

Assume you have an elderly population of 100,000 people; 10,000 have diabetes and 30,000 have cholecystitis. In the population 3,000 have both diseases if the diseases are not correlated but occur together with a frequency that follows simple probability laws. The probability of having both diseases equals the probability of having diabetes (0.1) and the probability of having cholecystitis (0.3); 100,000 × 0.3 × 0.1 = 3,000 with both diseases.

Let us now assume that 40% of patients with cholecystitis and 60% of diabetes patients become hospitalized. We then expect the following to be hospitalized:

Among the 7,000 with diabetes alone 60% will be hospitalized (4,200). Among those with cholecystitis alone 40% are hospitalized (27,000 × 0.40 = 10,800). For those with both diseases (3,000) we expect that they have a probability of being hospitalized either for one disease or the other. The number of people being hospitalized would then be

$$3,000 \times 0.4 + (3,000 - 1,200) \times 0.6 = 2,280$$

or the probability of being hospitalized for this group is 0.4 + 0.6 − 0.4 × 0.6 = 0.76.

Seventy-six percent of the 3,000 with both diseases become hospitalized, more than the 40 or 60% of those with either one of the two diseases.

Since having more than one disease will mean a higher probability of being hospitalized, these patients will constitute a larger fraction of hospital patients than they do in the population.

Mendelian Randomization

Results from large case–control or follow-up studies have sometimes been difficult to replicate in randomized trials. Observational studies on vitamin C, beta-carotene, and other vitamins have shown results that could not be replicated in randomized trials. These findings have been taken to indicate serious flaws in non-experimental epidemiology. We have to accept that it is difficult to estimate the effect of something that is closely correlated to many other habits that influence health without being able to randomize the exposure.

In some cases we may be able to use nature's own randomization process using the design known as *Mendelian randomization* or *Mendelian Deconfounding*. The design takes its name from Mendel's laws stating that hereditary traits are determined by pairs of genes of maternal and paternal origin that separate and reunite during reproduction. These pairs of genes, alleles, separate independently of other genes (if they are not close to each other on the chromosome) during this process. We have received the hereditary traits as part of a random process during the time of conception and we may use this randomness when designing our study.

The Mendelian randomization principle was first discussed by Katan in 1986 [3] at a time when it was a concern if cholesterol-lowering drugs would lead to cancer. Data did show a strong correlation between low cholesterol levels and cancer, but that could be a result of *reverse causation* if a not yet diagnosed cancer consumed cholesterol or reduced appetite. Genetic factors controlling cholesterol could be used to solve the problem of the causal direction (Fig. 21.3).

If the causal mechanism is as in Fig. 21.3 we would expect to see an association between genetic factors and cancer. If the association between low cholesterol and cancer is due to reverse causation (Fig. 21.4) we will not expect to see an association between the genetic factors and cancer, unless we stratify on cholesterol levels (adjust for cholesterol).

Fig. 21.3 Causal links
between genetic factors and
cancer

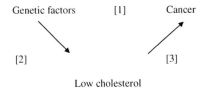

Fig. 21.4 No causal links
between genetic factors and
cancer

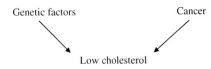

Fig. 21.5 No causal links
between genetic factors and
cancer

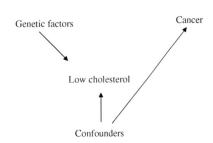

If the association between low cholesterol and cancer is due to confounding (Fig. 21.5) we will not expect to see an association between the genetic factors and cancer, unless we stratify on cholesterol levels.

The basic idea in Mendelian randomization is that we compare associations between different genotypes and the disease [1], although we believe the causal link of interest is given by the exposure (for example, cholesterol). For this to work we need to have a strong causal link between the genotype and the intermediate phenotype [2]. We call the genotype an "instrumental" variable for the phenotype of interest. If we have no direct link from the genotype to disease [1] then the entire genotypic effect is mediated by the phenotype [2+3]. If [1] presents a causal link, the association we see need not be related to the exposure (the phenotype) (Fig. 21.6).

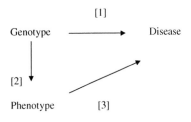

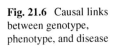

Fig. 21.6 Causal links
between genotype,
phenotype, and disease

We are estimating [1] but we are interested in [3], and using that strategy is similar to what we do in the randomized trial when we analyze data according to the "intention to treat" principle given by the randomization. It is not the randomization in itself that causes an effect, only the exposure that follows randomization.

By analyzing the association between the genotype and the outcome one avoids reverse causation since the genotype was present before the cancer (was present at the time of conception). Confounding should not be a problem because the genotype was allocated by a random process independently of factors that may affect the phenotype.

Even in the situation where the stated conditions are fulfilled the design may be flawed. The genotype may influence the phenotype. Slow metabolizers of alcohol may, for example, drink less than fast metabolizers. The genotype under study may be in disequilibrium with other genetic factors that impact disease risk. There may be other compensating factors that modify the effect, and the gene expression may be modified by factors that operate early in life (epigenetic changes).

Several observational studies have shown that a low intake of a vitamin B called folate or folic acid carries an increased risk for delivering a child with neural tube defect (NTD). It is believed that intake of folate reduces the level of homocysteine and could inhibit the closure of the neural tube and lead to NTD.

Two randomized trials [4] did strongly support that folate can reduce the prevalence at birth of NTD. These trials included people who did not receive the preventive factor and some children were therefore born with NTDs that could have been prevented. The randomized trial bypassed the problem that intake of folate correlates with many other factors (especially dietary factors). These other factors could be responsible for the preventive effect, but this confounding could also have been avoided in a Mendelian randomization study. People with the variant of the MTHFR gene who had high levels of homocysteine received this gene variant independently of other genetic or lifestyle factors as part of a random process. Mothers with the gene variant should have a higher risk of getting a child with an NTD than other women. The gene variant in fathers should not play a direct role since the father does not transmit homocysteine to the child during pregnancy, and these predictions seem to be corroborated by data. Due to the randomization process we would not expect women with the gene variant (they would not know about this) to have exposures to folic acid that differ from women without the gene variant. Using these principles may have replaced a randomized trial that had serious side effects for some.

References

1. Baastrup PC, Schou M.. Prophylactic lithium. Lancet 1968;1(7557):1419–1422.
2. Berkson J. Limitations of the application of fourfold table analysis to hospital data. Biomet Bull 1946;2:47–53.
3. Katan MB. Apolipoprotein E isoforms, serum cholesterol and cancer. Lancet 1986;i:507–508.
4. Czeizel AE. Primary prevention of neural-tube defects and some other major congenital abnormalities. Recommendations for the appropriate use of folic acid during pregnancy. Paediatr Drugs 2000;6:437–449.

Chapter 22
Sources of Error in Genetic Epidemiology

The effort to understand the link between genetic variants and human health and behavior has a good theoretical background as a high heritability has been demonstrated for a large number of traits.

However, there are a number of caveats that need to be considered when incorporating the results of genetic tests into epidemiologic analysis.

Multiple Testing

The enormous advances in genetic technology over the last few years have made it possible within a reasonable budget to go from studying a handful of gene variants to as many as one million per sample on thousands of individuals. The downside of this development is that any given study may be overwhelmed with *false positive findings* due to *multiple testing*. Tests of a million SNPs would be expected to generate 50,000 SNPs showing $P < 0.05$ by chance alone. This problem is magnified when subgroup analyses are performed as is done routinely, i.e., stratifying for sex, age, SES, etc., without clear a priori hypotheses. New analytic approaches to adjusting for multiple comparisons such as using the false discovery rate can assist in minimizing to a reasonable number the signals that require additional investigation. Eventually replications in well-defined, large, independent samples are central to dealing with these challenges, and currently the replications required often involve tens of thousands of individuals.

Not only the exposure side (genotypes) has contributed to the multiple testing problem, but also the outcome side (health, diseases, behaviors). It can be tempting to use the 1 million genetic markers one has obtained on a large sample of individuals to test for possible associations with the wide range of outcomes that often are available on such cohorts. This can be meaningful for well-defined traits with substantial heritability, but in some areas of behavioral research genetic variants are linked to "downstream behaviors," e.g., one type of behavior on a single occasion or a very specific type of behavior or vaguely defined behaviors. Such "downstream" behaviors are very likely to fluctuate over time and therefore have a much lower heritability than reliably constructed and validated measures such as personality type.

J. Olsen et al., *An Introduction to Epidemiology for Health Professionals*,
Springer Series on Epidemiology and Health 1, DOI 10.1007/978-1-4419-1497-2_22,
© Springer Science+Business Media, LLC 2010

It seems premature to try to link specific genetic variants to very specific behaviors with unknown heritability at a time when we are struggling to learn how to interpret genetic findings on valid behavioral phenotypes that can be measured reliably.

Population Stratification

Selection of the control group is often one of the biggest challenges in epidemiologic research and also in studies of genetic variants where differences in ethnic or racial background can create confounding in cohort and case–control studies of unrelated individuals – the so-called *population stratification*. The practical importance of this potential bias has been questioned, at least in non-Hispanic white populations of European descent where proper epidemiologic case–control methods have been used, but can be substantial in mixed populations. However, also in studies including both northern and southern Europe, population stratification can produce misleading results. For example, gene variants that show a north–south gradient (e.g., ApoE-4 or genes for lactose intolerance) will seem to be associated with height and skin color because there is also a north–south gradient in Europe in height and skin color. Population stratification can be removed by matching on ethnic/ancestral background, restricting studies to highly homogeneous populations and by using family-based controls. In addition, the large numbers of markers now being used allow for marker-based definitions of ancestry which may become far more accurate than self-identified ancestry and can be used itself to define matches in the case and control populations.

Laboratory Errors

Errors can occur in any area of scientific investigation, and genetics is no exception. Laboratory testing is only as reliable as the samples accurately reflect their biological origins. Mishandling and mislabeling can result in the wrong sample attached to the "right" data set. Sampling also may rely on accurate family histories so that non-paternity (and in an age of egg and embryo donation, non-maternity) and adoption must be considered and included in data collection to ensure that biological relationships are as stated. In the wet laboratory itself there is some imprecision of measurement that may be platform or sample dependent. When the DNA quality or quantity is suboptimal (especially in the use of archival samples not collected specifically for use in genotyping) the results may have some degree of inaccuracy that can escape detection. Case and control DNA, or infant and parent DNA, may come from different biological sources (blood spots on infants versus peripheral blood or saliva on parents, for example), and the behavior of DNA in genotyping assays is partly dependent on its origin and processing. In some cases of very limited DNA quantities amplification technologies may increase the amount of DNA available, but amplification is often non-homogeneous and can result in genotype failures or inaccuracies (for example, allele drop-out where one variant in a genotype fails to amplify and the other does turning a heterozygote into an apparent homozygote). The assays themselves may have noise in them that can result in inaccurate scoring. There are a variety of checks that can be applied to the genotype data to assist in using only data that are accurate but when millions of SNPs are scored on thousands of samples some degree of error is inevitable. Checks can include ensuring that Mendelian relationships fit with genotype data and that *Hardy–Weinberg equilibria* (HWE) are within accepted norms (with the caveat that HWE may be violated in case samples when the marker under study is strongly associated with the phenotype of interest. However, control samples failing to meet HWE suggest data errors). Occasionally Mendelian failures may be due to true allele loss in the case of copy number variants or de novo deletion events. Finally, minimum standards for the percent of samples that genotype successfully are also usually applied with some boundary line below which the marker is considered unusable. It is usually wise to mix cases and controls on analysis plates (currently assays are typically done using 96, 384, or 1, 536 well plates with each well holding one person sample) to avoid systematic errors related to plate effects. And in the end any positive results should be validated by repeating the assay using an alternative technology, using nearby SNPs to obtain similar results, and repeating in independent samples for true replication.

Chapter 23
Sources of Error in Clinical Epidemiology

Within the field of clinical epidemiology bias is always a concern and the field is plagued by studies which have not taken this into account. Lack of insights in problems caused by confounding by indication, differential misclassification of exposure, differential misclassification of outcome, and selection bias have resulted in premature claims of causality. However, it is fair to say that during the last decade there has been a growing awareness of the problems, but it is still too easy to find many examples of a suboptimal study design where bias has led to wrong results.

Confounding by Indication

Cholecystectomy is one of the most common surgical procedures. In Sweden there were 30,000 such operations annually during the 1970s. The number has decreased since then and there are now about 12,000 annually. As mentioned in Chapter 9 confounding by indication is an issue when evaluating the introduction of laparoscopic cholecystectomy compared to traditional surgery, as the non-complicated cases are more likely to be subjected to a laparoscopic procedure, thus causing bias when postoperative complications and duration of hospital stay are outcomes to be compared.

Concerns have also been raised that this operation will have long-term negative consequences such as an increased risk for colorectal and/or pancreatic cancer [1, 2]. Given the high numbers of such operations even a small effect would be of interest from a public health perspective. There are underlying potential biological mechanisms which give some credence to such a concern; a continuous flow of bile, due to the absence of a reservoir function of the gallbladder, could be a carcinogenic when the bile is not diluted by food intake. Moreover, a number of case–control studies dealing with the etiology for colorectal and pancreatic cancers published in the 1970s, 1980s, and early 1990s consistently demonstrated that a history of cholecystectomy was associated with an increased risk for both cancer forms.

J. Olsen et al., *An Introduction to Epidemiology for Health Professionals,*
Springer Series on Epidemiology and Health 1, DOI 10.1007/978-1-4419-1497-2_23,
© Springer Science+Business Media, LLC 2010

Furthermore, for colorectal cancer this association was most pronounced for right-sided colonic cancer, which according to some authors further strengthened the hypothesis since bile would be less diluted in the right side of the colon compared to the left side, but some were aware of the potential problem of detection bias. Abdominal symptoms from a not yet diagnosed cancer could lead to diagnostic work-up followed by a cholecystectomy if a diseased gallbladder was found. Such a scenario was more likely to be present for a right-sided colonic cancer than for a left-sided which then could be the underlying explanation for the findings described above. Most authors dealt with this problem by excluding cholecystectomies performed within a year prior to a diagnosis of either colorectal or pancreatic cancer. However, population-based register studies from Scandinavia have demonstrated that an association between cholecystectomy and both cancer forms exists up to 5 years after operation followed by no associations. Thus, the exclusion of cholecystectomies 1 year after operation may not be enough. The concerns of adverse long-term effects following the results of previous studies may be misplaced and underline the need for collaboration between epidemiologists and clinicians.

Differential Misclassification of Outcome

Vasectomy has repeatedly been suspected as a long-term risk factor for prostate cancer especially in northern America. Prostate cancer is, however, a disease where the diagnostic intensity is of major importance in descriptive epidemiology and may also be a concern in analytical studies. One of the first studies which explored the potential association was a case–control study where the medical history in 220 men with prostate cancer was compared to two different control groups, 571 non-cancer controls and 960 cancer controls using data from the hospital system [3]. Using non-cancer controls showed a fivefold excess risk of prostate cancer and a 3.5 risk when other cancer controls were used. The magnitude of a risk was unrelated to time after vasectomy, but the authors pointed out that the association was stronger among men more likely to have been under intensive medical surveillance, indicating that differential misclassification could be an issue. This was further explored in two cohort studies, one of husbands of nurses [4] and the second in health professionals [5], both with prostate cancer as an outcome with prospectively collected data on vasectomies. In the first study there were 96 cases of prostate cancer and in the second 300 cases. In both studies the authors demonstrated a significant excess risk of 50 and 60%, respectively, also for severe cases of prostate cancer. The presence of a higher point estimate among more severe cases was used by the authors as an argument against differential misclassification of the outcome as an explanation for their results. The authors justified their hypothesis by describing potential underlying biological mechanisms, an altered immune response for sperm antigens and/or a diminished prostate fluid secretion as a result of a vasectomy.

However, the most likely explanation for these results is differential misclassification; prostate cancer may have been diagnosed differentially among exposed and unexposed. Individuals with a history of vasectomy are more likely to undergo diagnostic procedures of the urogenital tract than others. Further credence for this explanation is given by the result from a register-based study from Denmark [6] where men subjected to a vasectomy showed no excess risk of prostate cancer during follow-up, a finding which is consistent with other study results published thereafter.

Differential Misclassification of Exposure

Induced abortion and its impact on the future risk of breast cancer is an example of another intervention where potential adverse events only can be assessed by observational studies. There is an underlying biological rationale for such an association. Differentiation of the breast parenchyma will start early during pregnancy and will be interrupted by an induced abortion and may create "fertile soil" for a later malignant transformation. There are animal models which give further support to such a mechanism. Differential misclassification of the exposure data (induced abortions) is, however, of major concern when studying this exposure.

The first large study of an association between induced abortion and breast cancer was a case–control study consisting of 845 cases of breast cancer and 961 control women from the USA with the focus of reproductive history [7]. The information was gathered by interviews with a high participation rate both among cases and controls. The authors demonstrated a 50% increased risk among women with a history of induced abortion compared to those without, and the highest risk was present among women with a history of induced abortion before the age of 18, with a relative risk of 2.5. There was no association between a history of spontaneous abortion and breast cancer, which was interpreted to support the idea as such pregnancies in most instances will not be associated with increased levels of pregnancy hormones. The authors were aware of the potential problem of differential misclassification, i.e., that cases and controls would have a different attitude to reveal sensitive information, such as a history of induced abortion. However, the authors had conducted a similar case–control study with cervical cancer as an outcome and in that study no association with abortion was found (4), which the authors used as an argument that differential misclassification did not explain the finding.

There was, however, reason to be concerned which was demonstrated by a Dutch study [8]. This study had a very similar design to the US study with 918 women with breast cancer and as many controls. The authors found a 90% increased risk among those with a history of induced abortion, but after stratifying on areas with a Roman Catholic population who were less likely to disclose a history of induced abortion the authors demonstrated that no such association existed outside the Roman Catholic area. Differential misclassification of exposure related to religious beliefs emerged as the most likely explanation for an association between breast cancer and induced abortion, a hypothesis given further credibility by the results from Scandinavian register-based studies [9].

Selection Bias

Randomized clinical trials have shortcomings in evaluating rare adverse events, and observational studies are the only alternative design. Selection bias is a concern and must be in the back of any investigator's mind. An illustrative example is what has happened after the introduction of *anti-TNF medications* 10 years ago for different inflammation disorders such as rheumatoid arthritis and Crohn's disease. These compounds represent a new biological class, and concerns were raised early on that they could adversely affect the immune system.

The first study which evaluated the risk of non-Hodgkin's lymphomas (NHL) in patients treated with these compounds demonstrated an excess risk for NHL following exposure to anti-TNF medication compared to exposures to other medications in patients with rheumatoid arthritis [10]. It is, however, a well-known fact that rheumatoid arthritis is associated with an excess risk of NHL, and this increased risk is strongly associated with inflammatory activity. Selection bias could therefore be an alternative explanation as candidates for this treatment will be those who have failed to respond to the previously available medications. These patients will consequently have been exposed to higher inflammatory activity over time compared to other patients with rheumatoid arthritis and thus have the highest risk for NHL. It is therefore reassuring that later follow-up studies of "normal" unselected patients with rheumatoid arthritis did not show any increased risk of NHL following exposure to anti-TNF therapy compared to other patients with rheumatoid arthritis with the same history of disease activity [11].

References

1. Lagergren J, Ye W, Ekbom A. Intestinal cancer after cholecystectomy: is bile involved in carcinogenesis? Gastroenterology 2001;121(3):542–547.
2. Ye W, Lagergren J, Nyrén O, Ekbom A. Risk of pancreatic cancer after cholecystectomy: a cohort study in Sweden. Gut 2001;49(5):678–681.
3. Rosenberg L, Palmer JR, Zauber AG, Warshauer ME, Stolley PD, Shapiro S. Vasectomy and the risk of prostate cancer. Am J Epidemiol 1990;132(6):1051–1055.
4. Giovannucci E, Tosteson TD, Speizer FE, Ascherio A, Vessey MP, Colditz GA. A retrospective cohort study of vasectomy and prostate cancer in US men. JAMA 1993;269(7): 878–882.
5. Giovannucci E, Ascherio A, Rimm EB, Colditz GA, Stampfer MJ, Willett WC. A prospective cohort study of vasectomy and prostate cancer in US men. JAMA 1993;269(7):873–877.
6. Lynge E. Prostate cancer is not increased in men with vasectomy in Denmark. J Urol 2002;168(2):488–490.
7. Daling JR, Malone KE, Voigt LF, White E, Weiss NS. Risk of breast cancer among young women: relationship to induced abortion. J Natl Cancer Inst 1994;86(21):1584–1592.
8. Rookus MA, van Leeuwen FE. Induced abortion and risk for breast cancer: reporting (recall) bias in a Dutch case-control study. J Natl Cancer Inst 1996;88(23):1759–1764.
9. Melbye M, Wohlfartht J, Olsen JH, Frisch M, Westergaard T, Helweg-Larsen K, Andersen PK. Induced abortion and the risk of breast cancer. N Engl J Med 1997;336(2):81–85.
10. Geborek P, Bladström A, Turesson C, Gulfe A, Petersson IF, Saxne T, Olsson H, Jacobsson LT. Tumour necrosis factor blockers do not increase overall tumour risk in patients with

rheumatoid arthritis, but may be associated with an increased risk of lymphomas. Ann Rheum Dis 2005;64(5):699–703.

11. Askling J, Baecklund E, Granath F, Geborek P, Fored M, Backlin C, Bertilsson L, Cöster L, Jacobsson LT, Lindblad S, Lysholm J, Rantapää-Dahlqvist S, Saxne T, van Vollenhoven R, Klareskog L, Feltelius N. Anti-tumour necrosis factor therapy in rheumatoid arthritis and risk of malignant lymphomas: relative risks and time trends in the Swedish Biologics Register. Ann Rheum Dis 2009;68(5):648–653.

Part IV
Statistics in Epidemiology

There are many good statistical textbooks on the market, and we refer readers to some of these textbooks when they need statistical techniques to analyze data or to interpret statistical results. This book will not provide even a short introduction to statistics.

Most epidemiologic studies are now analyzed by using powerful statistical models that require software and computers. The ease of using these tools is, however, troublesome unless you are familiar with the conditions these methods rest upon. We strongly advocate that data analyses always start with simple tabulations of key variables. Looking at data stratified by the key exposures, outcomes, and confounders will often provide the information you seek, and if results differ much from what you get from simple tabulations after extensive computer massage you need to check your computations carefully. Your modeled results may be true, but more often they will not be. Model assumptions may be grossly violated or the results may be due to coding mistakes, inappropriate handling of missing data, or other errors that may not be easily detected in the output you get. Furthermore, most statistical models used to analyze complex data rest on assumptions that are rarely fulfilled. Tests of violations of these assumptions are usually weak, and lack of evidence against model assumptions is weak evidence in favor of these assumptions. This is especially true in smaller data sets.

Statistical models rest upon assumptions on how data interact. This usually concerns whether they interact in an additive or multiplicative way. We rarely have reason to believe data should follow either of these two interaction patterns. Nonetheless, if deviations from these model assumptions are small, they often work reasonably well.

Additive Model

We talk about additive models if the absolute effect measure (e.g., rate difference) remains the same across all strata and if combined effects are obtained by adding risks for the main factors. In the simplest form, *additive data* will look like Table 23.1.

Table 23.1 Additive model

Confounder/ modifier	Exposure	Incident rate (per 10,000 person-years)	Rate difference (per 10,000 person-years)
–	+	10	
	–	5	5.0
+	+	20	
	–	15	5.0

Note: A potential effect modifier need not be a confounder.

The absolute increase in incidence rate remains the same with 5 per 10,000 person-years when stratifying on a third variable (another determinant of the disease, a possible confounder/effect measure modifier). We conclude that different levels of this third variable do not (in this data source) modify our estimated effect measure (the rate difference).

If this was written in incidence rate ratio (IRR) terms, using as the reference category those unexposed to C and E, where C is the confounder and E the exposure, we would get the following:

$(IRR_{EC} - 1)$	=	$(IRR_E - 1)$	+	$(IRR_C - 1)$
$(20/5 - 1)$	=	$(10/5 - 1)$	+	$(15/5 - 1)$
$(4 - 1)$	=	$(2 - 1)$	+	$(3 - 1)$

Again we can see that the expected effect on the additive scale is equal to the observed effect. There is no effect measure on the additive scale.

Multiplicative Model

Most scientific papers focus on the *multiplicative model,* since the effect estimates are often relative estimates (OR, RR, or IRR). By changing just one line of results in the table above (the additive model), we can make the associations multiplicative. If so, the table would look like Table 23.2.

Table 23.2 Multiplicative model

Confounder/ modifier	Exposure	Incidence rate (per 10,000 person-years)	IRR
–	+	10	
	–	5	2.0
+	+	30	
	–	15	2.0

Note: A potential effect modifier need not be a confounder.

The association is called multiplicative because the incidence rate ratio of the combined exposure (E and C) is the multiplication of the incidence rate ratios or relative risks of the single exposures.

IRR_{EC}	$=$	IRR_E	$\times$	IRR_C
(30/5)	$=$	(10/5)	$\times$	(15/5)
6	$=$	2	$\times$	3

We can see that the observed effect measure is as we would expect, and therefore there is no interaction on the multiplicative scale.

Statisticians talk about *interaction* when the stratum-specific effect measures differ more than we would expect – more than random variation could justify. If in Table 23.1 we estimated the IRR we would find an interaction between the exposure and the confounder since we were assessing the interaction on the multiplicative scale instead of the additive scale: $IRR_{C-} = 10/5 = 2.0$ and $IRR_{C+} = 20/15 = 1.33$ (2.00 is different from 1.33 – at least in a larger sample).

Similarly, if we estimate the IRD from Table 23.2 we get the following:

IRD_{C-}	$=$	$(10-5)_{\text{person-years}}^{-1}$	$=$	$5_{\text{person-years}}^{-1}$
IRD_{C+}	$=$	$(30-15)_{\text{person-years}}^{-1}$	$=$	$15_{\text{person-years}}^{-1}$

The two absolute risk estimates (IRD) differ; there is an effect modification on the additive scale. In the presented situations classification of interactions is measure specific (and we should therefore talk about *effect measure modification*), since the interaction will disappear when applying the effect measure that best describes the data.

Data need not follow an additive model or multiplication model. The association could, for example, be more than multiplicative as illustrated in Table 23.3:

Table 23.3 More than multiplicative association

Confounder/ modifier	Exposure	Incidence rate (per 10,000 person-years)	IRR
–	+	10	
	–	5	2.0
+	+	60	
	–	15	4.0

We should then present stratum-specific results rather than a combined measure. Epidemiologists talk about effect measure modification either in the statistical sense (as the statisticians talk about interaction) or in the biological sense. For example, two exposures may impact the same receptor. Or one exposure may block the effect of another if they are both metabolized by the same enzymes and the effect stems from their metabolites. Most complex metabolic routes are not expected to lead to simple additive or multiplicative associations, and in general there are no strong reasons to believe biological effects would follow any of these two models. This does not mean they are useless. We just have to accept that they produce average measures that do not fully provide all information.

To check how your variables interact you should start out by stratifying data. This should be done not only in order to study effect measure modification and/or confounding, but, perhaps most importantly, to get an idea about the data structure and identify coding errors.

Stratification is also a powerful and easily understood method of controlling for confounding. If you wanted to study whether the intake of carrots protects against lung cancer you would want to make comparisons among people who have the same expected background risk of lung cancer had the exposed not been exposed. We know that lung cancer risk varies with sex, race, age, and smoking habits and also with exposure to certain types of air pollution. We would like to make comparisons within a stratum that could look like Table 23.4.

Table 23.4 One stratum in a stratified analysis

Sex	Race	Age	Smoking	Air pollution	Carrots	Observation time	Lung cancer
M	AI	50–54 years	10–14 cig.	High	Yes	t_+	a_+
					No	t_-	a_-

Having done that, we would like to summarize the IRR we get from each stratum to a common estimate given we see no interaction/effect measure modification.

Mantel–Haenszel's formulas for analyzing stratified data [1] have served epidemiologists well for decades. Despite common belief that the formulas have only historical interest we present them below. The formulas can be easily applied by anyone using a simple hand calculator. Most often, we used logistic regression, Cox regression, and other models because the computer will do the calculations for you. In addition, the stratification method has limitations – especially in smaller data sets. For example, if you have 2 sex groups, 8 age groups, and 3 air pollution levels, the data would be divided into $2 \times 8 \times 3 = 48$ strata. The study would need to be large enough to provide sufficient information within all 48 strata. The following methods will exclude strata that have no exposed or no unexposed, no diseased or no non-diseased within each stratum. These strata with marginal zeros provide no information to the analyses although they may provide important information for your inference. Accepting a more complicated statistical model allows you to make use of all data.

Imagine a follow-up study reconstructed after an incident of food poisoning. Exposure could be exposure to ice cream. Data lay-out could be as in Table 23.5.

In the analysis the focus is upon the a cell, exposed with the disease. For this a cell we calculate the expected value, had the combined disease experience for the stratum been applied to all exposed in that stratum:

Table 23.5 Stratified analyses for Mantel–Haenszel analysis	Stratum	Exposure	D	$\overline{D}$	n
	j	$+$	a_j	b_j	n_{j+}
		$-$	c_j	d_j	n_{j-}
			D_j	$\overline{D}_j$	n_j

$$E_{(a_j)} = \frac{D_j n_{j+}}{n_j}$$

Then we calculate the variance of the a cell and our estimate of the relative risk, RR_{MH}:

$$Var(a_j) = \frac{n_j + n_j - D_j \overline{D}_j}{n_j^2(n_j - 1)}$$

We then combine results from all strata to get a combined estimate of RR:

$$RR_{MH} = \frac{\sum a_j \frac{n_{j-}}{n_j}}{\sum c_j \frac{n_{j+}}{n_j}}$$

and the χ^2 test of the difference between the disease risk among exposed versus non-exposed is (now summarized over all strata)

$$\chi^2 = \frac{(\sum a_j - \sum E(a_j))^2}{\sum Var(a_j)}$$

In a study on incidence rates the table will look like Table 23.6.

Table 23.6 Stratified analysis of rate data	Stratum	Exposure	D	Person-time
	j	$+$	a_j	t_{j+}
		$-$	c_j	t_j
			D_j	T_j

The expected value of the a_j cell becomes

$$E_{(a_j)} = \frac{D_j t_{j+}}{T_j}$$

The variance of the a cell is

$$Var(a_j) = D_j \frac{t_{j+} t_{j-}}{T_j^2}$$

$$IRR_{MH} = \frac{\sum \frac{a_j t_{j-}}{T_j}}{\sum \frac{c_j t_{j+}}{T_j}}$$

and the χ^2 test of the null hypothesis of no association between the exposure and the disease is, like before,

$$\chi^2 = \frac{\left(\sum a_j - \sum E(a_j)\right)^2}{\sum Var(a_j)}$$

Reference

1. Mantel N, Haenszel W. Statistical aspects of the analysis of data from retrospective studies of disease. J Natl Cancer Inst 1959;22:719–748.

Chapter 24
P Values

In the past, much emphasis was put on the so-called *significance testing*. The investigator assumed a null hypothesis stating no association between the exposure and the disease (usually the real hypothesis would be the opposite of the null hypothesis). Then he/she would calculate a *P value*. The *P* value would indicate the probability of getting the data he/she found or data that were even further away from the null hypothesis (the no-effect value), given the null hypothesis was true (and other conditions). If this *P* value was below a given level (often <0.05) it was said that the finding was statistically significant and the null hypothesis was rejected as a likely explanation of the data.

There are several reasons why this practice should be abandoned. First, the interpretation requires a randomized trial. For a non-randomized study we would have to add a sentence like "If this study was randomized, then. ..." Clearly this poses a severe limitation on the *P* value interpretation in non-randomized studies to a level where it is almost meaningless.

Second, most decisions should not be forced to follow a simple decision rule unless it is absolutely necessary, and classifying results as significant or not significant lends itself to such a simple decision process. Significance testing was developed as a decision tool in mass production where it may serve a quality control purpose well. In public health we would almost never base a decision on a simple statistical rule, and only rarely will this be the case in the decision process following a randomized trial, although it may be so if the randomized trial is the only evidence we have.

We have the four outcomes of a decision based upon a *P* value testing a *null hypothesis* (H_0) in Table 24.1.

Table 24.1 Type 1 and type 2 errors

H_0	H_0 accepted	H_0 rejected
True	OK	Type 1 error
False	Type 2 error	OK

As seen, two of the four outcomes are wrong. The risk of a *type 1 error* is set by the significance level (often 0.05). The risk of accepting a false H_0, that the effect

J. Olsen et al., *An Introduction to Epidemiology for Health Professionals*,
Springer Series on Epidemiology and Health 1, DOI 10.1007/978-1-4419-1497-2_24,
© Springer Science+Business Media, LLC 2010

of the exposure is overlooked, is a function of several conditions. The *type 2 error* is high if the study is small or if the effect is small. It depends on the significance level of testing and the sample size. The power of the study equals (1 − risk of type 2 error). The power indicates the probability of finding a true effect of a given size and with a given sample size.

It is difficult to see why we should accept to base our decision on a *P* level only and few would probably do so. *P* values are still computed, but more attention is given to estimates of association and their confidence limits, although confidence limits often indicate only part of the uncertainty related to the measure of effect. Uncertainty is also related to residual confounding and other types of bias. Opinions are based on the combined available evidence. Good studies carry more weight than poor studies. Simple replication studies carry less weight than studies that bring the hypothesis to a more critical test. When to take action furthermore depends on the consequences of doing nothing versus doing something. There is no *P* value substitute for common sense and critical thinking but brain surgery may be needed to remove *P* values from epidemiologic papers. The most serious flaw in using *P* values is to infer that there is no association if the *P* value is 0.05 or higher. Absence of evidence is not evidence for absence of an effect! A failure to recognize this simple fact has caused much harm to many innocent people.

Further, uncertainty is related to residual confounding and/or various types of bias. Opinions are based upon the combined evidence available. Good studies have more weight than poor studies. Simple replication studies carry less weight than studies that put the hypothesis to a more critical test. When to take action furthermore depends upon the consequences of doing nothing versus doing something. There is no substitute for common sense and critical thinking.

The multiple comparison problem is a problem related to presenting only statistically significant results to the reader. If you generate a data source at random with a large number of exposures and a disease, then test the associations between the disease and this exposure and then calculate *P* values. These *P* values will fall on a 45° line as illustrated in Fig. 24.1.

The number of significant associations (that all are generated by randomness in this example) is determined by the number of tests we perform, and since these associations are spurious they tend not to be replicable in other studies. We would like to avoid presenting these associations, but unfortunately, there is no simple way

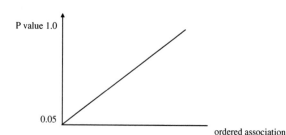

Fig. 24.1 *P* value plot of ordered associations

of doing this. Simple correction factors, like the Bonferroni correction that approximately reduces your significance level by the number of tests you perform (if you do 10 tests your level of significance should not be 0.05 but 0.005), aims at keeping the risk of producing one or more spurious significant results less than 0.05. Unfortunately, it is seldom that simple. First of all, this is not how serious epidemiologists analyze and report results. Second, the simple Bonferroni correction is often wrong. The principles for analyzing data are to follow a specific a priori hypothesis and then evaluate if your data supported the hypothesis or not. You would like to know how much you have to adjust your prior belief in the hypothesis you had given the data. Furthermore, when you identify an association you should try to see how robust it is. In your analyses you will try to see if you can make the association go away by adjusting for confounding or other sources of error. You will check if the association is consistent in relevant strata, etc. You will of course also report non-significant associations in your paper. Proper analyses of epidemiologic data have nothing to do with uncritical testing for a large number of associations and only reporting significant *P* values. Remember that any source of information will only modify your prior belief in the association, to make this belief stronger or weaker.

Chapter 25
Calculating Confidence Intervals

Confidence intervals provide more information than a P value and do not in the same way tempt readers to make simplified conclusions; ideally they provide a range of effect measures that are "acceptable" given the data. If the null value (RR, IRR $= 1$; RD, IRD $= 0$) is not among these, the result is statistically significant, and the no-effect hypothesis is not a likely explanation for the data. Many would find that this description is too vague, but a more precise description would have to take into consideration a number of assumptions that are beyond this text. To calculate confidence limits for the risk ratio or the relative risk (RR) we need to calculate the variance of the log of the Mantel–Haenszel estimated relative risk.

The formula for the variance of the RRs is

$$\text{Var(ln (RR}_{\text{MH}})) = \frac{\sum \dfrac{D_j n_{j+} n_{j-}}{(n_j^2 - a_j c_j)/n_j}}{\sum \dfrac{a_j n_{j-}}{n_j} \sum \dfrac{c_j n_{j+}}{n_j}}$$

The 95% confidence limits (indicated by RR$_L$ and RR$_{UL}$) will be

$$\text{RR}_{\text{LL}} = e^{\ln (\text{RR}_{\text{MH}}) - 1.96\sqrt{\text{Var(ln (RR}_{\text{MH}}))}}$$
$$\text{RR}_{\text{UL}} = e^{\ln (\text{RR}_{\text{MH}}) + 1.96\sqrt{\text{Var(ln (RR}_{\text{MH}}))}}$$

The value 1.96 provides a P value of 0.05 in a standard normal distribution of $\sqrt{X^2}$ values and we take the square root of the variance to get standard deviation. The variance formula for the Mantel–Haenszel odds ratio (OR$_{\text{MH}}$) is

$$\text{Var(ln (OR}_{\text{MH}})) = \frac{\sum A_j X_i}{2 \left(\sum A_i\right)^2} + \frac{\sum (A_i Y_i + B_i X_i)}{2 \left(\sum A_i \sum B_i\right)} + \frac{\sum B_i Y_i}{2 \left(\sum B_i\right)^2}$$

where $A_j = (a_j d_j/n_j)$, $X_j = (a_j + d_j)/n_j$, $B_j = (c_j b_j/n_j)$, and $Y_j = (c_j + b_j)/n_j$.
And the two confidence limits are (like before)

J. Olsen et al., *An Introduction to Epidemiology for Health Professionals*,
Springer Series on Epidemiology and Health 1, DOI 10.1007/978-1-4419-1497-2_25,
© Springer Science+Business Media, LLC 2010

$$OR_{LL} = e^{\ln(OR_{MH})-1.96\sqrt{Var(\ln(OR_{MH}))}}$$
$$OR_{UL} = e^{\ln(OR_{MH})+1.96\sqrt{Var(\ln(OR_{MH}))}}$$

For the Mantel–Haenszel incidence rate ratio we get

$$Var(\ln(IRR_{MH})) = \frac{\sum\left(\dfrac{D_j t_j + t_{j-}}{T_j^2}\right)}{\left(\sum \dfrac{a_j t_{j-}}{T_j}\right)\left(\sum \dfrac{c_j t_{j+}}{T_j}\right)}$$

and the two confidence limits are (like before)

$$IRR_{LL} = e^{\ln(IRR_{MH})-1.96\sqrt{Var(\ln(IRR_{MH}))}}$$
$$IRR_{UL} = e^{\ln(IRR_{MH})+1.96\sqrt{Var(\ln(IRR_{MH}))}}$$

Although most confidence intervals in epidemiology have no precise meaning they are still useful as a familiar measure of part of the uncertainty inherent in our measures of association. They at least remind us that other effect estimates are also acceptable explanations of the data.

Epilogue

The laws of nature are to be discovered, not to be invented, as Pierre Louis Maupertuis stated in the nineteenth century. These laws of nature deal with the many different factors that impact our health. The laws are often complex and involve many different component causes, and they will only reveal themselves when you combine data from many people. For that reason epidemiology is a population science.

As explained in this book, population studies (epidemiologic studies) are saddled with problems and limitations, and do not think that all the examples provided in this book can be generalized to all other situations. Still, epidemiologic studies are, and will remain, the most important studies if your goals are to prevent disease, improve health, and provide the best possible health care.

History has shown that epidemiology, with all its problems and shortcomings, has provided much useful information that has improved our life expectancy and quality of life [1]. It is therefore necessary for health professionals to at least have some knowledge about the methods epidemiologists use and their limitations. Carefully done epidemiologic studies will not only provide new and valid information but will also identify false beliefs and misconceptions. Nothing more than common sense is perhaps needed to do epidemiologic research, but common sense is a remarkably rare trait that needs to be stimulated by training and education. If this book makes you aware of what you do not know you are on your way to becoming a better epidemiologist.

Reference

1. Holland WW, Olsen J, Florey CDV. The Development of Modern Epidemiology. Oxford University Press, Oxford, 2007.

Index

Breinigsville, PA USA
19 May 2010
238318BV00006B/28/P